CDN

Study Guide

2025-2026

Certified Dialysis Nurse Certification Exam Review + 500 Q&A and Practice Tests, Proven Strategies to Ace the Exam

Chris Moore

Disclaimer

The information provided in this book is for educational and informational purposes only. While every effort has been made to ensure the accuracy and reliability of the content, the author and publisher do not make any warranties, expressed or implied, regarding the accuracy, completeness, or usefulness of the information contained herein.

This book is not intended to serve as professional advice, and readers should not rely solely on the information provided without seeking professional guidance tailored to their specific needs or circumstances.

The author and publisher shall not be held responsible for any errors or omissions, or for any damages arising from the use or reliance on the information presented in this book, including but not limited to direct, indirect, incidental, or consequential damages.

Table of Contents

Introduction:

In today's fast-paced digital world, speed and performance are no longer optional. They are vital to user satisfaction, business success, and even SEO rankings. Whether you're running an e-commerce website, managing a global media platform, or providing online services, the speed at which your content loads can make or break the user experience. The internet is inherently complex, with the physical distance between servers and users contributing to latency and slow load times. This is where Content Delivery Networks (CDNs) come into play, offering a powerful solution to overcome the challenges of content delivery.

CDNs have become a cornerstone of modern web infrastructure, ensuring that content—ranging from static files like images and videos to dynamic web applications and APIs—loads quickly, reliably, and securely, no matter where the user is located. As businesses expand globally, the need to optimize the delivery of digital content to users in different geographic regions has grown exponentially. CDNs allow content to be cached and served from a network of servers strategically placed around the world, ensuring that users always get the fastest access to the content they need.

In this guide, we will explore the world of Content Delivery Networks in depth. This is not just a technical manual for engineers or IT professionals; it's an all-encompassing learning resource that aims to demystify CDNs for anyone seeking to understand how they work and why they matter. Whether you're a business owner, a developer, a network engineer, or simply someone interested in the technology behind the fast internet we experience every day, this guide will take you through the core concepts, use cases, strategies, and hands-on techniques required to master CDNs.

To start, let's take a step back and look at the fundamental question: *What is a CDN?*

At its core, a Content Delivery Network is a system designed to efficiently deliver content to users by distributing it across a network of servers that are geographically distributed. These servers are called edge servers, and they store cached copies of the content—whether it's a video, an image, a website, or even an API call. When a user makes a request for that content, the CDN routes the request to the server closest to the user, significantly reducing the time it takes for the content to reach them. By minimizing the distance between the user and the server, CDNs reduce latency and improve load times, leading to a better user experience.

In practical terms, CDNs can dramatically reduce the burden on a website's origin server, improve website performance, enhance security, and provide a more consistent user experience across various devices and network conditions. The benefits of using a CDN are numerous, especially when dealing with high-traffic websites or applications that need to deliver content to users across the globe. CDNs help websites scale, ensuring that no matter how many users access the content, the delivery remains fast and reliable.

The early days of the internet were defined by relatively slow, geographically isolated server connections. A request for a website from a user in Europe, for instance, would have to travel all the way to the server in the United States, often experiencing significant delays. As the internet grew, so did the need for faster content delivery. Over time, CDNs evolved to address this challenge by deploying servers in multiple locations, reducing the distance content had to travel, and improving load times. The development of CDNs represented a major leap forward in internet performance and scalability.

However, as the demands of internet traffic continue to evolve, so too must CDNs. Today, CDNs are more than just tools for caching static content. They play a crucial role in delivering dynamic content, ensuring real-time data processing, and even providing security features such as DDoS protection and secure delivery of sensitive information. With the advent of edge computing, CDNs are also becoming platforms for running serverless functions, processing data closer to the user, and enabling ultra-low-latency interactions. This has opened new possibilities for applications ranging from online gaming to interactive video streaming, e-commerce, and IoT.

As businesses and users increasingly expect faster, more reliable web experiences, CDNs have grown into a foundational technology for modern internet architecture. Content providers now rely on CDNs not only for speed but for the resilience they offer. When one server or data center goes down, a well-configured CDN can reroute traffic to other operational servers, ensuring continuous uptime. This built-in redundancy and fault tolerance make CDNs indispensable in a world where downtime can lead to lost revenue, customer dissatisfaction, and damage to brand reputation.

Moreover, CDNs are an essential tool for improving the security of web traffic. They can help mitigate distributed denial-of-service (DDoS) attacks by distributing the incoming traffic across a network of edge servers. If one server is overwhelmed by malicious traffic, the CDN can absorb the attack and block malicious requests, safeguarding the origin server from being taken offline. Additionally, many CDNs offer SSL/TLS encryption at the edge, ensuring secure delivery of content without putting undue load on the origin server.

The global nature of the internet means that users from all corners of the world expect seamless access to content, regardless of their location or device. As a result, CDNs are critical for global businesses, media companies, e-commerce sites, and any service that requires high-performance web delivery. Whether users are accessing your website from New York, Tokyo, or Nairobi, a CDN ensures that content is delivered quickly and efficiently, optimizing the experience for each individual based on their location and the available network conditions.

However, despite the numerous benefits, CDNs are not a silver bullet. They come with their own set of challenges. For example, correctly configuring a CDN requires an understanding of caching rules, content expiration, and the need to balance load across multiple servers. Also, CDNs are not always suited for every type of content or use case. While they excel in delivering static content like images, stylesheets, and videos, they may not be the best fit for all dynamic content, especially if it requires frequent updates or personalized delivery. Additionally, the reliance on third-party CDN providers means that businesses must trust these external services with their critical content delivery, which can raise concerns about privacy and data security.

In the following chapters, we will dive deep into these topics, unpacking the underlying technologies that power CDNs and exploring the best practices for using them effectively. You will learn about the anatomy of a CDN, the role of edge servers, caching mechanisms, and how content is routed across the network to ensure the fastest possible delivery. You will also gain hands-on knowledge on how to configure a CDN for different use cases, optimize performance, and troubleshoot common issues that arise in real-world deployments.

We will also explore the advanced features and capabilities of CDNs, such as real-time content optimization, edge computing, and the integration of serverless functions. These innovations are transforming the way CDNs operate, enabling them to deliver faster, smarter, and more flexible solutions for modern applications.

To further enrich your learning, we will take a closer look at industry-specific use cases and success stories, drawing from the experiences of large-scale companies that rely on CDNs to power their digital services. From global media companies like Netflix to tech giants such as Amazon and Google, we'll explore how CDNs have helped these companies scale, innovate, and deliver world-class user experiences.

Finally, as you master the fundamentals of CDNs, we'll examine where the technology is headed in the future. With the growing importance of edge computing, artificial intelligence (AI), and machine learning, CDNs are becoming even more powerful, efficient, and adaptive to the needs of modern users. We'll discuss these emerging trends and provide you with insights into how to stay ahead of the curve as CDNs continue to evolve.

By the end of this guide, you'll have a comprehensive understanding of CDNs, from their basic principles to advanced deployment strategies. Whether you're a developer, network engineer, or business decision-maker, you'll be equipped to leverage the power of CDNs to optimize performance, enhance security, and improve the overall user experience for your online services.

The world of CDNs is constantly changing, but one thing remains certain: in the digital age, delivering content quickly and efficiently is not just a convenience—it's a necessity. So, let's begin this journey to unlock the full potential of Content Delivery Networks and explore how they can help you achieve faster, more reliable, and more secure content delivery in an increasingly connected world.

Understanding CDNs: An Overview

In the modern digital ecosystem, the demand for faster, more reliable internet experiences has never been higher. Whether it's a website loading in mere seconds, streaming video content without buffering, or an e-commerce platform delivering seamless user interactions, speed has become a cornerstone of user satisfaction. But what enables this speed? How can a website or service ensure its content reaches users across the globe quickly and efficiently? The answer, in large part, lies in the use of **Content Delivery Networks (CDNs)**.

A Content Delivery Network is a system of distributed servers designed to deliver web content, applications, and services to users with high availability and performance. Instead of relying on a single server to handle all requests, a CDN distributes content across a network of geographically dispersed servers, called **edge servers**, which are positioned closer to the end-users. This architecture allows CDNs to provide faster content delivery, reduce latency, and offer improved fault tolerance and scalability for web applications and websites.

To understand the value and impact of CDNs, it's important to break down what they do, how they work, and the role they play in the broader context of internet performance. Let's take a deeper look at the fundamentals of CDNs, starting with the core concepts behind their design and operation.

A **Content Delivery Network (CDN)** essentially acts as an intermediary between the origin server (the server where the original content is hosted) and the end-users (the people or devices requesting that content). When a user requests a resource, such as a web page, an image, or a video, the CDN determines which of its edge servers is closest to the user and delivers the requested content from there. By reducing the physical distance between the user and the content, CDNs significantly reduce the time it takes for content to travel across the internet—this is often referred to as **latency**. The closer the server is to the user, the faster the content is delivered, which enhances user experience.

CDNs use a combination of intelligent routing algorithms and caching mechanisms to ensure that content is delivered from the most appropriate server in the network. When a request for content is made, the CDN first checks to see if it already has a cached copy of that content on the edge servers. If the content is available in cache, it is delivered immediately, and the user's request is handled by the nearest server. If the content is not cached, the CDN fetches it from the origin server, caches it on the edge server, and serves it to the user. This process not only reduces load times but also helps reduce the load on the origin server, as repeated requests for the same content are served by the edge servers rather than the central origin.

A CDN's network is made up of multiple **edge servers**, which are strategically placed in data centers around the world. The number and distribution of these edge servers depend on the scale of the CDN and the geographical reach required. Global CDNs, such as Cloudflare, Akamai, and AWS CloudFront, have thousands of edge locations across different regions and continents, enabling them to serve content quickly to users no matter where they are. By distributing content across multiple locations, CDNs also provide redundancy—if one server or data center fails, another can step in and continue delivering the content, ensuring uninterrupted service.

One of the primary functions of a CDN is to **cache content**. When a user requests a particular resource for the first time, the CDN fetches it from the origin server and caches it at the nearest edge server. The cached version of the content is stored in memory for a specific period of time, known as the **Time to Live (TTL)**. TTL determines how long the cached content will remain valid before it is considered outdated and must be refreshed from the origin server. Different types of content have different TTL settings; for example, static content like images or JavaScript files may have longer TTL values, while dynamic content (such as personalized web pages or user data) may be cached for much shorter periods, or not cached at all.

CDNs are not only effective for caching static content like images, videos, or stylesheets but also for accelerating the delivery of **dynamic content**. Dynamic content is typically generated on-the-fly based on user interactions or data from backend systems, such as personalized web pages, live data, or search results. Traditionally, dynamic content was challenging to serve through CDNs because it changes frequently and cannot be easily cached. However, modern CDNs have developed advanced techniques to handle dynamic content, such as caching dynamic assets for short periods, intelligently fetching data from the origin server, or even using **edge computing** to process some requests at the edge of the network, closer to the user. This ensures that even complex web applications can benefit from the performance gains provided by CDNs.

Another important benefit of using a CDN is the **improvement of website reliability and availability**. In the traditional setup, if the origin server goes down or experiences high traffic, users may be unable to access the content. A CDN mitigates this risk by replicating content across multiple edge servers. If one server fails or becomes overloaded, the CDN can automatically route the request to the next available edge server. This ensures that users can still access the content without interruptions, even during periods of high traffic or unexpected server failures. CDNs also help with **scalability**, allowing websites to handle spikes in traffic without overloading the origin server or compromising performance.

Security is another crucial advantage of using CDNs. By acting as a middle layer between users and origin servers, CDNs can provide a level of protection against various types of cyberattacks. One of the most common threats faced by websites is **Distributed Denial-of-Service (DDoS)** attacks, in which a network of compromised devices floods a website with an overwhelming amount of traffic, causing it to become slow or even crash. CDNs can help mitigate DDoS attacks by distributing the traffic across multiple servers, which makes it more difficult for attackers to target any one server. Many CDNs also offer **SSL/TLS encryption** at the edge, ensuring that data transmitted between the user and the CDN is secure. Additionally, some CDNs provide Web Application Firewalls (WAFs), which help protect websites from malicious traffic, SQL injection attacks, cross-site scripting (XSS), and other threats.

The impact of CDNs on **web performance** is perhaps one of the most significant benefits they offer. As websites and applications become more resource-intensive and media-heavy, the demands on network performance have grown. Users expect faster load times and smooth experiences, whether they are viewing a high-definition video, browsing an image gallery, or interacting with a real-time application. Slow load times can lead to user frustration, increased bounce rates, and even lost revenue, especially for e-commerce businesses. A CDN can dramatically reduce the time it takes for content to load, making websites feel more responsive and improving the overall user experience. Faster websites are also rewarded by search engines, as Google and other search engines factor page load speed into their ranking algorithms.

The use of CDNs is not limited to traditional websites. CDNs are increasingly being adopted in various industries for a range of applications. In the **video streaming industry**, CDNs are essential for delivering high-quality video content to viewers with minimal buffering. Services like Netflix, YouTube, and Vimeo rely on CDNs to ensure that users can stream videos without interruptions, regardless of their location or device. CDNs help optimize video quality by delivering adaptive bitrate streaming, which adjusts the video quality based on the user's internet connection speed, ensuring smooth playback even in low-bandwidth environments.

In **mobile applications**, CDNs play a crucial role in improving the speed and reliability of content delivery to users. Mobile networks can be less reliable than wired networks, and users expect content to load quickly, even on slow or spotty connections. CDNs help mobile apps deliver images, videos, and data to users in real-time, while also reducing the load on the mobile app's backend servers. This can improve the overall mobile user experience, reduce latency, and increase user retention rates.

For businesses with a global reach, CDNs are indispensable for **global website optimization**. Whether your website is serving users in New York, London, Sydney, or Tokyo, a CDN ensures that content is delivered quickly to all corners of the world, without requiring users to wait for distant servers to respond. This has become especially important in an age where more and more businesses are expanding internationally, and a global presence online is critical for success.

However, CDNs are not without challenges. One of the main issues businesses face when implementing CDNs is **cost**. While CDNs can significantly improve performance, they also come with a price tag. The cost of using a CDN is often determined by factors like data transfer volume, the number of edge servers, and the type of content being delivered. For small businesses or websites with low traffic, this may not be a significant concern. But for large-scale enterprises with high-volume traffic or complex content delivery needs, CDN costs can add up quickly. It's important for businesses to carefully evaluate their CDN provider options and determine the most cost-effective solution based on their specific needs.

Another challenge is **configuration and maintenance**. Setting up a CDN requires an understanding of how caching works, how to configure content delivery rules, and how to manage the distribution of content across multiple servers. If not configured correctly, a CDN can end up delivering stale or outdated content to users, resulting in poor user experiences. It's also crucial to monitor the performance of the CDN regularly to ensure that it is functioning optimally and providing the expected performance benefits.

Despite these challenges, the advantages of using a CDN far outweigh the drawbacks for most businesses and applications. By improving website performance, increasing reliability, enhancing security, and offering scalability, CDNs are an essential part of modern web infrastructure. As the internet continues to evolve and content delivery needs become more complex, the role of CDNs will only grow in importance, helping businesses deliver a faster, more secure, and more reliable experience to users around the globe.

In conclusion, a Content Delivery Network is an indispensable tool for delivering fast, reliable, and secure web content across the globe. Whether you're a small business, a large enterprise, or a service provider, understanding how CDNs work and leveraging their power can make a significant difference in your ability to meet user expectations, scale your operations, and compete in a global digital marketplace. By optimizing the delivery of your content, CDNs help ensure that your website, application, or service is not only fast but also resilient, secure, and ready to handle the demands of a constantly connected world.

Study Strategies for Mastering Content Delivery Networks (CDNs)

Mastering Content Delivery Networks (CDNs) is essential for anyone aiming to excel in modern web technologies and digital performance optimization. Whether you're a developer, network engineer, or IT professional, understanding how CDNs function and how to optimize their usage can significantly boost your skill set and career prospects. The following comprehensive study strategies will guide you through mastering CDN concepts effectively, offering methods that promote understanding, retention, and practical application.

1. **Start with the Basics: Build a Solid Foundation**

Before diving into the complexities of CDNs, it is crucial to understand the fundamental concepts that underpin CDN technology. This includes understanding how data is transferred across networks, how the internet works, and the key terms used in CDN architectures, such as edge servers, origin servers, caching, and latency. Without grasping these foundational concepts, it will be difficult to understand more advanced CDN optimization techniques.

A good starting point for beginners is to familiarize yourself with how content is typically delivered across the internet. Research key internet protocols such as HTTP/HTTPS, DNS (Domain Name System), TCP/IP, and CDN-specific protocols. Understanding these will provide context for how CDNs enhance performance by routing traffic through the most optimal paths.

Once you're comfortable with the basics of how data moves across networks, it becomes easier to understand the role of CDNs in this process. The key concepts of CDNs—such as load balancing, caching, geolocation, and how they contribute to faster content delivery—should become your core focus. This knowledge will be foundational for your journey into more specialized CDN optimization strategies.

2. Break Down Complex Topics into Digestible Sections

CDNs are a multifaceted technology, encompassing a wide variety of technical components. It can be overwhelming to study the entire system at once. To improve retention, break down the information into smaller, manageable chunks. You can organize your study material into categories such as:

- CDN Architecture and Components (Edge Servers, Origin Servers, Caching)
- CDN Performance and Optimization Strategies
- CDN Security Considerations
- CDN Use Cases and Industry Applications
- Real-World Case Studies

This will make the subject matter less daunting and help you focus on mastering one aspect of CDN technology before moving on to the next. Each time you master a category, the next section will build upon what you already know. This approach allows you to gradually increase your depth of knowledge and confidently move from one complex topic to the next.

3. Use Real-World Examples and Case Studies

One of the most effective ways to solidify your understanding of CDNs is by studying real-world applications and case studies. By examining how large organizations like Netflix, Amazon, and

YouTube use CDNs to improve user experience, you'll gain practical insights into how CDNs are used in production environments.

Look for industry-specific case studies where CDNs have been implemented to solve real-world problems. For example, you can learn how gaming companies use CDNs to handle massive traffic during game launches, or how e-commerce platforms optimize CDN strategies to manage high volumes of traffic during seasonal sales like Black Friday or Singles' Day.

By relating the theoretical concepts you've learned to tangible examples, you'll better understand how to implement CDN technology in various contexts. Additionally, reading case studies from diverse industries—ranging from e-commerce to media streaming to SaaS—will broaden your understanding of CDN's capabilities and applications.

4. Hands-on Learning and Labs

CDN technologies can often be understood better through hands-on experience rather than through theory alone. Setting up and configuring a CDN yourself will give you a more practical understanding of how CDNs work. Start with small projects like integrating a simple CDN into a website or testing performance improvements on static resources like images and JavaScript files.

Many CDN providers such as Cloudflare, Akamai, Amazon CloudFront, and Fastly offer free tiers or trial periods. These platforms typically have comprehensive documentation and tutorials to help you get started. By experimenting with different CDN configurations, you can observe firsthand how caching, content delivery, and optimization settings affect website performance.

If you're working with a development environment, you could simulate different scenarios such as traffic spikes, load balancing, and regional content delivery, all of which will give you insight into how CDNs handle real-world traffic.

Building your practical knowledge is critical in preparing for exams or certifications on CDN technologies. Try to incorporate lab exercises where you set up a CDN to test things like caching behavior, edge server performance, and the impact of dynamic versus static content delivery. This type of hands-on practice will make you more confident in applying CDN technologies to your projects.

5. **Study CDN Performance and Optimization Strategies**

Once you understand the architecture of CDNs, dive deeper into performance optimization techniques. This is where the real power of CDNs is unlocked. Focus on key optimization strategies such as:

- **Caching Strategies:** Learn about cache-hit vs. cache-miss scenarios and understand how TTL (Time-to-Live) affects content delivery. Understand how CDNs cache content at the edge servers and how to configure cache control headers for maximum efficiency.

- **Latency Reduction:** Explore ways to reduce latency using CDNs. This could involve learning how to configure geo-distribution of edge servers, choosing the optimal CDN provider for your audience, or implementing HTTP/2 and QUIC for faster data transfer.

- **Adaptive Bitrate Streaming:** Learn how video streaming platforms like Netflix and YouTube utilize adaptive bitrate streaming. This allows CDNs to deliver the highest quality video stream based on the viewer's internet connection, ensuring smooth playback even in variable network conditions.

- **Pre-fetching and Content Pre-positioning:** Understand how CDNs can predict user requests and pre-fetch content to edge servers before users request it, thus reducing load times for frequently accessed resources.

- **Load Balancing and Traffic Routing:** Study how CDNs intelligently route traffic based on factors such as server load, network congestion, and the geographic location of the user. Understanding how to implement efficient load balancing strategies will help you optimize performance.

By mastering CDN optimization techniques, you'll not only understand how to use a CDN but also how to make it work more efficiently and effectively for different kinds of content and traffic.

6. **Focus on Security and Threat Mitigation**

CDNs are not just about performance; they also play a crucial role in web security. Learning how to use a CDN for security purposes will add a valuable skill to your repertoire. Many CDN providers offer built-in security features such as DDoS protection, SSL/TLS encryption, Web Application Firewalls (WAF), and bot mitigation tools.

Understanding how CDNs mitigate common internet security threats is crucial, especially if you're working in industries that handle sensitive data. Pay attention to how CDNs help with:

- **DDoS Protection:** Learn how CDNs absorb malicious traffic by distributing the load across their global network, preventing attacks from overwhelming your origin servers.

- **Secure Data Delivery:** Understand how CDNs facilitate the delivery of secure content using SSL certificates and HTTPS, ensuring that sensitive data is encrypted during transit.

- **Bot Protection and Rate Limiting:** Investigate how CDNs use edge servers to detect and mitigate bot traffic, ensuring that only legitimate users can access your website.

7. Take Advantage of CDN Documentation and Resources

One of the best resources for learning about CDNs is the documentation provided by CDN providers. Every major CDN service has detailed documentation on how to implement and optimize its services. Some examples include:

- **Cloudflare's Knowledge Base**: A treasure trove of articles and tutorials on CDN configuration, security features, and performance optimization.

- **AWS CloudFront Documentation**: In-depth guides for integrating AWS CloudFront with other AWS services, caching techniques, and performance tuning.

- **Akamai Developer Tools**: A set of resources for advanced CDN users, including APIs, optimization techniques, and troubleshooting guides.

In addition to provider documentation, there are numerous online resources such as blogs, YouTube tutorials, and forums where professionals share insights on best practices, configurations, and troubleshooting techniques.

Participate in online communities such as Stack Overflow, Reddit, or specialized forums dedicated to CDN technologies. Asking questions and sharing your experiences with others will deepen your understanding and expose you to real-world challenges and solutions.

8. Utilize Practice Exams and Quizzes

If you're preparing for certifications or exams related to CDN technology, practice exams can be a very helpful way to assess your readiness. There are many resources available online with practice questions on CDN architecture, performance optimization, security, and troubleshooting. Make use of these quizzes to test your understanding of key concepts before taking the actual exam.

Review the explanations for each answer, especially for those you get wrong. This will help you identify areas that require more focus and attention. Repeated practice with these quizzes will also help reinforce the material and increase your chances of success.

9. Collaborate with Peers and Experts

Another highly effective study strategy is to collaborate with others who are also learning or working with CDNs. Group study sessions, online meetups, and discussion groups allow you to exchange knowledge, troubleshoot problems together, and learn from others' experiences.

If you're in a professional environment, consider pairing up with colleagues or attending workshops and webinars where you can ask questions and engage in discussions with experts in the field. Additionally, many CDN providers offer training programs, certifications, and forums where you can ask questions and learn from experts in the field.

10. Stay Updated with Industry Trends and Emerging Technologies

The world of CDNs is constantly evolving. New technologies, features, and strategies are emerging all the time, and staying updated with industry trends will help you remain competitive. Follow industry blogs, attend conferences (virtually or in person), and keep an eye on any new research papers or white papers released by major CDN providers or industry organizations.

Emerging technologies like **Edge Computing**, **Serverless Architectures**, and **AI-Driven Performance Optimization** are transforming the CDN landscape. By learning about these innovations, you'll be well-equipped to tackle the next generation of CDN technologies.

By following these comprehensive study strategies, you'll be able to master CDNs in a structured and effective way. Whether you're learning for personal development, certification, or to apply CDN technologies in your career, these strategies will help ensure a deep understanding of CDNs and the tools needed to optimize them. Keep learning, experimenting, and adapting to the rapidly changing digital landscape!

Study Tips from Experts for Mastering CDNs

Mastering Content Delivery Networks (CDNs) involves both theoretical understanding and hands-on experience. To help you approach your study effectively, here are expert study tips that will guide you through the process:

1. Understand the Fundamentals Before Diving into Advanced Topics

- **Tip**: Don't rush into advanced CDN features like edge computing or security optimizations before understanding the core concepts.
- **Why it works**: Mastering the basics, such as how CDNs work, the difference between edge and origin servers, and caching mechanisms, is crucial. Without this foundation, advanced topics might feel overwhelming and disconnected.
- **Action**: Spend the first few weeks reviewing core concepts like caching, DNS routing, and latency optimization. Use diagrams and analogies to visualize the CDN architecture.

2. Break Down Complex Concepts into Smaller Chunks

- **Tip**: Break large topics, such as CDN architecture or security protocols, into smaller, digestible pieces. Study them one by one rather than trying to grasp everything at once.
- **Why it works**: Large concepts can be overwhelming. Breaking them down helps you focus on specific areas and prevents burnout.
- **Action**: Start with a chapter like "How CDNs Work" and break it down into sub-topics: edge servers, caching, geolocation, DNS, etc. Understand each before moving on to the next.

3. Leverage Hands-On Learning

- **Tip**: Set up a real-world CDN integration (even a basic one) and experiment with it. The best way to understand a CDN is by actually using one.

- **Why it works**: Hands-on experience is invaluable when it comes to learning technologies like CDNs. It helps solidify theoretical knowledge and gives you a practical understanding of the challenges and configurations involved.

- **Action**: Sign up for a CDN trial (e.g., Cloudflare, AWS CloudFront) and implement it on a personal or test website. Try caching static files, configuring DNS settings, and testing performance improvements.

4. Practice with Real-World Scenarios

- **Tip**: Study CDNs through the lens of real-world use cases such as media streaming, e-commerce, and global content delivery.

- **Why it works**: Understanding how CDNs are applied in various industries gives you a broader context and makes the technology more relevant and memorable.

- **Action**: Review case studies of CDN use, such as how Netflix handles high demand for streaming, or how e-commerce sites like Amazon use CDNs to optimize global performance.

5. Learn the Language of CDNs and Networking

- **Tip**: Familiarize yourself with key terms such as TTL (Time to Live), cache-hit, cache-miss, purging, edge computing, and DNS routing.

- **Why it works**: Understanding the terminology helps you read and comprehend documentation more effectively. It also ensures that you can communicate clearly with others when discussing CDNs.

- **Action**: Create flashcards for key CDN concepts and terms. Review these regularly to reinforce your understanding.

6. Stay Current with Industry Trends

- **Tip**: Follow industry blogs, forums, and news related to CDNs, networking, and cloud services. Technologies like edge computing and AI integration are rapidly evolving in the CDN space.

- **Why it works**: The CDN landscape is continuously changing with new innovations. Staying updated ensures you understand the latest trends and technologies, making you more adaptable and knowledgeable.

- **Action**: Subscribe to blogs like Cloudflare's Blog, AWS CloudFront Blog, or other industry-specific sources to keep up-to-date.

7. Use Visual Aids to Reinforce Understanding

- **Tip**: Draw diagrams or use tools like Canva or Lucidchart to visualize CDN architectures and processes.

- **Why it works**: Visualizing complex systems helps in understanding the flow of data, the relationship between servers, and the interaction of various components (e.g., caching, DNS, geolocation).

- **Action**: Create diagrams for CDN architecture, including the relationship between origin servers, edge servers, and clients. Include aspects like content routing, TTL, and security features.

8. Set a Study Schedule and Stick to It

- **Tip**: Structure your study time and set realistic goals for each session.
- **Why it works**: Consistency is key when mastering a technical subject like CDNs. A study schedule helps you stay on track, retain information, and avoid overwhelming yourself.
- **Action**: Create a weekly study plan. For example, Monday could be dedicated to reading theory, Tuesday to watching tutorials, Wednesday to hands-on practice, and Thursday for reviewing case studies.

9. Join Study Groups or Online Communities

- **Tip**: Join forums or study groups (e.g., Stack Overflow, Reddit's r/sysadmin or r/networking) to discuss CDN concepts and learn from others' experiences.
- **Why it works**: Interacting with peers allows you to clarify doubts, share insights, and stay motivated. Explaining concepts to others can also reinforce your understanding.
- **Action**: Participate in discussions about CDNs, ask questions when you encounter challenges, and share your experiences with setting up CDNs or optimizing performance.

10. Use Multiple Learning Resources

- **Tip**: Don't rely solely on one source. Combine textbooks, online tutorials, documentation, and videos to get a more well-rounded understanding of CDNs.

- **Why it works**: Different resources explain the same concepts in various ways, and you might find one explanation resonates more with you.

- **Action**: Use official documentation from CDN providers (Cloudflare, Akamai, AWS) and supplement it with YouTube tutorials, courses on Udemy or Coursera, and blog posts.

11. Test Yourself Regularly

- **Tip**: Take quizzes, practice exams, or write summaries of what you've learned.

- **Why it works**: Self-testing reinforces what you've learned and highlights areas where you need more review.

- **Action**: At the end of each study session, write a short summary or test yourself with questions like "What is TTL in CDN caching?" or "How does DNS routing work in a CDN?"

12. Focus on Problem-Solving, Not Just Theory

- **Tip**: Rather than just memorizing definitions, focus on solving problems related to CDN configuration, troubleshooting, and performance optimization.

- **Why it works**: CDNs are practical technologies, so understanding how to apply theory to solve real-world issues is critical.

- **Action**: Work through practical labs or real-world scenarios, such as diagnosing performance issues on a website that uses a CDN or configuring caching rules for a specific use case (e-commerce vs. video streaming).

Bonus Tip: Be Patient and Persistent

- **Tip**: CDNs can be complex, and mastering them takes time and practice. Don't get discouraged by setbacks or difficult concepts.
- **Why it works**: Persistence is key to mastering technical subjects. Even when things feel difficult, consistent effort will pay off.
- **Action**: Celebrate small wins along the way—like configuring a simple CDN or understanding caching mechanisms—and remember that learning is a gradual process.

Study Strategies for Mastering CDNs

Studying Content Delivery Networks (CDNs) requires a combination of theoretical knowledge, practical experience, and continuous learning. Whether you're preparing for a certification, a project, or simply deepening your expertise, the following study strategies will help you approach the subject in an organized and effective way.

1. Start with the Basics: Lay a Strong Foundation

- **Strategy**: Begin by thoroughly understanding the **fundamentals of networking and web performance** before diving deep into CDNs. CDNs build upon concepts like HTTP/HTTPS, DNS, and caching, so knowing these topics inside-out is crucial.
- **Action**:

- Study basic networking concepts like IP addressing, routing, and DNS.

- Understand HTTP/HTTPS protocols, including request-response cycles, headers, and status codes.

- Familiarize yourself with basic caching mechanisms (browser caching, server-side caching, and CDN caching).

- **Why this works**: A strong foundational understanding of how the internet works and how data flows will make advanced CDN topics easier to grasp and apply.

2. Break Down the Content into Manageable Sections

- **Strategy**: Divide the study material into smaller, digestible pieces. Focus on one concept or sub-topic at a time, and avoid trying to learn everything at once.

- **Action**:

    - Tackle each chapter or section of your study guide step-by-step.

    - Break larger topics into mini-topics (e.g., in CDN architecture, study edge servers, origin servers, and caching separately before combining them).

- **Why this works**: Breaking down complex topics reduces cognitive load and prevents feeling overwhelmed. Small, focused study sessions also improve retention and comprehension.

3. Combine Theory with Hands-On Practice

- **Strategy**: Implement what you learn by setting up your own CDN configurations. Theoretical knowledge is essential, but practical experience is what truly solidifies your understanding.

- **Action**:
  - Set up a basic CDN on your personal website or a test environment using providers like Cloudflare, AWS CloudFront, or KeyCDN.
  - Experiment with caching rules, load balancing, and DNS settings.
  - Test different content types: static (images, scripts) and dynamic (API responses).
- **Why this works**: Hands-on learning accelerates comprehension. By applying theory to real-world scenarios, you gain a deeper understanding of CDN setups, issues, and optimizations.

4. Use Real-World Case Studies

- **Strategy**: Study CDN use cases in various industries (e-commerce, media streaming, SaaS, etc.) to understand how CDNs solve specific challenges in different contexts.
- **Action**:
  - Research case studies from companies that heavily rely on CDNs, such as Netflix, Amazon, or Spotify.
  - Pay attention to how CDNs handle performance optimization, content caching, and security (e.g., DDoS protection).
- **Why this works**: Real-world examples provide practical insights and help you connect abstract concepts to tangible applications. It also broadens your understanding of how CDNs are used across different sectors.

5. Review and Reinforce Key Concepts Regularly

- **Strategy**: Regularly review and reinforce what you've learned to avoid forgetting key concepts. Spaced repetition is a powerful technique for mastering technical material.

- **Action**:
  - Create **flashcards** for CDN terminology (e.g., TTL, cache-hit, purging) and key concepts (e.g., edge servers, content routing, load balancing).
  - Use tools like Anki or Quizlet to quiz yourself periodically on these terms.
  - Write summaries or "cheat sheets" for each chapter that highlight important points.

- **Why this works**: Spaced repetition boosts memory retention and ensures that key concepts stay fresh in your mind. Regular review helps identify areas where you need more focus.

6. Visualize Complex CDN Architectures

- **Strategy**: Visualizing content delivery networks helps clarify how different components (edge servers, origin servers, cache, DNS, etc.) interact and how data flows.

- **Action**:
  - Draw diagrams of the CDN architecture, including how content is routed from the origin server to edge servers and ultimately to the user.
  - Use diagramming tools like Lucidchart, Draw.io, or even pen-and-paper to sketch different configurations (e.g., for load balancing, caching, etc.).

- **Why this works**: Visual aids are powerful tools for reinforcing your understanding. Seeing how each part of the CDN architecture fits together makes the technology easier to grasp and troubleshoot.

7. Simulate Real-World Problems

- **Strategy**: Practice solving real-world problems you might encounter when deploying or managing CDNs. Simulating scenarios like performance degradation, security issues, or cache misconfigurations will prepare you for real-world challenges.

- **Action**:

  - Set up a scenario where the cache is misbehaving (e.g., stale content or cache misses) and troubleshoot using tools like **CDN provider dashboards** or **browser dev tools**.

  - Simulate a DDoS attack and explore how your CDN mitigates the attack using its security features.

  - Test how changing Time-to-Live (TTL) affects cache behavior and performance.

- **Why this works**: Simulating real-world issues helps build problem-solving skills and prepares you for practical challenges when implementing CDNs in production environments.

8. Use Online Resources and Communities

- **Strategy**: Engage with online communities, read blogs, and watch tutorials to deepen your understanding and stay updated with CDN technology trends.

- **Action**:

  - Follow industry blogs like **Cloudflare Blog, AWS CloudFront Blog**, or **Akamai Blog** for the latest trends and case studies.

  - Participate in **Reddit threads, Stack Overflow discussions**, and **forums** to learn from others' experiences and share your own.

- o Watch YouTube tutorials or courses on platforms like Udemy or Coursera.
- **Why this works**: Learning from experts in the field, engaging with peers, and staying up-to-date with industry trends gives you a competitive edge. It also provides different perspectives on solving problems.

9. Teach What You Learn

- **Strategy**: Teaching others, whether in a formal setting or informally, helps reinforce your own knowledge and uncover gaps in your understanding.
- **Action**:
  - o Create blog posts or YouTube videos explaining CDN concepts.
  - o Share your knowledge with friends, colleagues, or study groups.
  - o Answer questions on forums like Stack Overflow or Reddit related to CDN topics.
- **Why this works**: Teaching is one of the best ways to learn. Explaining complex topics to others forces you to articulate your thoughts clearly and ensures you understand the material deeply.

10. Plan for Exams or Certifications

- **Strategy**: If you're preparing for a certification or exam, structure your study plan to cover all topics systematically and take practice tests to gauge your progress.
- **Action**:

- Use resources like the **AWS Certified Solutions Architect – Associate** exam guide or similar certifications (e.g., Akamai or Cloudflare certifications) to align your study plan.
- Take **practice quizzes** to simulate exam conditions and identify weak spots.

- **Why this works**: A structured approach helps you prioritize study material based on exam objectives. Practice exams build confidence and highlight areas that need improvement.

11. Stay Organized and Manage Your Time

- **Strategy**: Use a study schedule to stay on track and avoid cramming. Breaking down study time into focused, manageable sessions helps you absorb more information effectively.

- **Action**:
  - Use a tool like **Trello** or **Notion** to organize your study tasks and track progress.
  - Set specific goals for each session (e.g., "Today I'll study DNS and CDN routing").
  - Avoid multitasking and set **study blocks** of 45-60 minutes with short breaks in between (the Pomodoro Technique).

- **Why this works**: Time management and organization help keep you motivated and productive. It also prevents procrastination and ensures consistent progress toward your goals.

Conclusion

Mastering CDNs requires a combination of **strong foundational knowledge**, **hands-on practice**, and **consistent reinforcement**. By breaking down the material, applying what you learn, and utilizing multiple study methods, you'll develop a deep and practical understanding of CDNs. With these study strategies, you can confidently tackle challenges in content delivery and stay ahead of the curve in a rapidly evolving field.

The Core Concepts of CDN Architecture: A Comprehensive Guide

Content Delivery Networks (CDNs) have become an indispensable technology for modern web applications, offering improved performance, scalability, and reliability. As more businesses move their services online and cater to a global user base, the need for efficient, high-speed content delivery is more critical than ever. Understanding the core concepts behind CDN architecture is essential for anyone working in web performance, networking, cloud services, or IT infrastructure. This article will dive deep into the key components of CDN architecture, breaking down each concept and exploring how they work together to deliver optimal web experiences.

The CDN Architecture Overview

At a high level, a CDN is a distributed network of servers strategically placed across various geographic locations. These servers are designed to cache and deliver content—such as images, videos, HTML files, and scripts—closer to the end user. The goal is to reduce latency, enhance content delivery speeds, and provide redundancy to ensure high availability even during traffic spikes or network failures.

The architecture of a CDN involves several key components and concepts that work together to deliver this functionality. These include **Edge Servers**, **Origin Servers**, **Caching Mechanisms**, **Load Balancing**, **Content Routing**, and **Geolocation**. Let's explore each of these core elements in more detail.

Edge Servers: The Frontline of Content Delivery

Edge servers are the backbone of a CDN. These servers are placed at strategic geographic locations to bring content closer to users. The term "edge" refers to the point where the user's request meets the network. Edge servers are positioned in data centers across various regions, creating a globally distributed network. When a user requests content, the CDN automatically routes that request to the nearest edge server. By serving content from these geographically distributed locations, CDNs can dramatically reduce latency and improve performance for users, especially those who are far away from the origin server.

The proximity of edge servers to end users is crucial for optimizing load times. For example, a user in New York accessing a website hosted in San Francisco will experience slower page loads compared to a user accessing the same website from a server located in New York. Edge servers store copies of static content, like images, videos, JavaScript files, and even HTML documents, making them readily available for quick delivery without having to retrieve the content from the origin server each time.

Edge servers also help offload traffic from the origin server, reducing its load and the amount of data that needs to be sent over long-distance links, which helps ensure a more efficient delivery system. Additionally, they provide fault tolerance; if one edge server goes down, the CDN can route traffic to another nearby edge server, preventing any single point of failure.

Origin Servers: The Source of Content

While edge servers are responsible for delivering cached content to users, origin servers are where the original content resides. Origin servers are typically the source of dynamic content or content that isn't cached at the edge servers. For example, the database-driven content of a website, such as personalized user data or product availability, is usually fetched from the origin server.

The role of the origin server in a CDN is to act as the authoritative source of content. When a user requests content that isn't cached on the edge server, the CDN will forward that request to the origin server to fetch the data. Once the content is retrieved, the edge server caches it for future requests, reducing the need to access the origin server repeatedly.

Origin servers are typically located in central data centers and can be optimized for processing dynamic requests or generating real-time content. Depending on the CDN configuration, the origin server may also handle security, authentication, or data consistency tasks.

In a well-optimized CDN setup, the origin server is shielded from heavy traffic loads and can focus on generating dynamic content or handling administrative tasks. By distributing traffic and caching static content at the edge, CDNs ensure that the origin server isn't overwhelmed by a large number of requests, especially during traffic surges.

Caching Mechanisms: Reducing Latency and Bandwidth Usage

Caching is one of the fundamental techniques employed by CDNs to speed up content delivery. The idea is simple: instead of fetching content from the origin server for every user request, content is stored locally on edge servers, so that subsequent requests can be served from the cache. This not only reduces the load on the origin server but also minimizes network congestion by reducing the number of long-distance data transfers.

There are different caching strategies and mechanisms in place for handling static and dynamic content. Here are some of the core caching concepts within a CDN architecture:

- **Cache Hits and Cache Misses:** A **cache hit** occurs when the content requested by the user is already available on the edge server. This means the request can be served directly from the cache, resulting in faster load times and less bandwidth usage. A **cache miss**, on the other hand, happens when the requested content isn't available on the edge server, so the CDN must fetch it from the origin server.

- **Time to Live (TTL):** TTL defines how long content remains cached on an edge server before it is considered stale and must be refreshed from the origin server. Short TTLs are often used for dynamic content or content that changes frequently, while long TTLs are used for static content that doesn't change often.

- **Cache Control Headers:** Content providers can control caching behavior by using HTTP headers like Cache-Control, Expires, or ETag. These headers instruct the CDN on how to cache content, whether it can be shared across multiple users, and how long it should be cached. This allows fine-grained control over content caching strategies.

- **Purging:** Caching is not a permanent solution; at some point, the cached content may need to be purged or updated. CDNs support content purging either based on the TTL or through manual invalidation, allowing users to refresh their content as needed.

By implementing effective caching mechanisms, CDNs can dramatically reduce latency, improve website load times, and save bandwidth for both content providers and end users.

Content Routing: Directing User Requests

Content routing is the process by which a CDN determines which edge server should handle a user's request. It ensures that user requests are routed to the optimal server based on a number of factors, such as geographic proximity, server health, load balancing, and network conditions. This is crucial for minimizing latency and improving overall user experience.

There are several methods that CDNs use for content routing:

- **Geolocation Routing:** This is one of the most common methods of content routing. When a user makes a request, the CDN determines their location (usually via IP address) and directs the request to the closest edge server, minimizing the physical distance the content has to travel. This reduces latency and improves load times.

- **Anycast Routing:** Anycast is a routing method that allows multiple edge servers to share the same IP address. When a user sends a request, the request is routed to the nearest edge server with that IP address. This can improve redundancy and fault tolerance, as requests are automatically routed to the closest server in case of failure or congestion.

- **Load Balancing:** To ensure that no single server is overwhelmed with traffic, CDNs use load balancing techniques to distribute user requests evenly across edge servers. This can be done by considering server capacity, current load, and server health. Load balancing ensures that content is served efficiently and that performance remains consistent even during traffic spikes.

- **Failover and Redundancy:** In the event that an edge server becomes unavailable, failover mechanisms can redirect requests to the next available server. This improves the reliability of content delivery and ensures high availability even in the event of server failure.

Effective content routing ensures that CDN services remain fast, resilient, and responsive, regardless of geographic location or server health.

Geolocation and Its Role in CDNs

Geolocation is a key component of CDN architecture that ensures content is delivered with minimal delay to users around the world. By determining the geographic location of the user and matching that location with the nearest edge server, CDNs can ensure that content is delivered with low latency. This is especially important in applications where speed is crucial, such as video streaming, gaming, e-commerce, and real-time communications.

Geolocation-based routing can significantly reduce the time it takes for data to travel between users and servers, as well as mitigate issues caused by network congestion, routing inefficiencies, or long-distance communication. Geolocation is also critical for personalized experiences, where user-specific content or language preferences are served from local servers based on the user's location.

In addition to reducing latency, geolocation also plays a key role in enabling **regional content restrictions**, **local compliance**, and **localized content delivery**. For example, CDNs can serve region-specific content, ensure compliance with regional data laws, and help companies target users with content tailored to their location.

Load Balancing: Optimizing Server Efficiency

Load balancing is another critical element in CDN architecture that ensures optimal use of resources, prevents bottlenecks, and improves overall system reliability. When many users access content simultaneously, load balancing ensures that the request traffic is distributed across multiple edge servers or across multiple data centers to avoid overloading any single server.

Load balancing works by monitoring the load on each server and redirecting requests based on real-time conditions. If one edge server is busy or underperforming, the CDN will automatically reroute requests to another server in a less congested location. This improves the responsiveness of the network and ensures that users receive content without delays, even during periods of high traffic.

Additionally, load balancing can help with **scalability**, allowing CDNs to handle sudden surges in traffic. Whether it's a holiday shopping season, a live-streaming event, or a viral content launch, CDNs are equipped to automatically scale resources to meet demand.

Conclusion

CDN architecture is a sophisticated, multi-faceted system designed to optimize the delivery of web content across the globe. By understanding the key components—**edge servers, origin servers, caching mechanisms, content routing, load balancing**, and **geolocation**—you can appreciate how these elements work together to provide fast, reliable, and scalable content delivery. As web traffic grows and user expectations increase, the role of CDNs will continue to be essential in ensuring that digital content is delivered efficiently, securely, and in a way that enhances the user experience.

Mastering these core concepts is essential for anyone working with or developing web technologies, as they form the foundation for creating performant, scalable, and resilient web applications. Whether you're involved in the development, management, or optimization of websites, understanding CDN architecture will equip you with the knowledge needed to tackle today's complex performance challenges.

The Core Concepts of CDN Architecture:

1. What does a CDN primarily aim to improve in terms of web content delivery?

   a) Security

   b) Content availability

   c) Speed and performance

   d) Data encryption

2. Which type of server in a CDN is responsible for storing the original, unmodified content?

   a) Edge server

   b) Origin server

   c) Proxy server

   d) Database server

3. What is the main role of an **edge server** in a CDN architecture?

   a) To store the original content

   b) To handle the database requests

   c) To cache content closer to end users

   d) To authenticate user requests

4. Which of the following is a key benefit of using edge servers in a CDN?

   a) Reduced storage requirements

   b) Reduced latency

   c) Increased origin server bandwidth

   d) Improved data encryption

5. How does a CDN improve website performance for users geographically far from the origin server?

   a) By compressing images

   b) By routing traffic through the nearest edge server

   c) By decreasing DNS query times

   d) By reducing the amount of content delivered

6. What is **Time to Live (TTL)** in the context of CDN caching?

   a) The time a file stays on the origin server

b) The maximum time a cached file remains in an edge server cache before being updated

c) The time it takes for a file to be delivered to the user

d) The lifetime of a DNS record

7. When a CDN server delivers content to a user from its cache, this is referred to as a:

a) Cache miss

b) Cache hit

c) Cache refresh

d) Cache purge

8. What is a **cache miss** in CDN terminology?

a) When content is served directly from the origin server

b) When the content is not available in the edge server's cache and needs to be retrieved from the origin server

c) When content is purged from the cache

d) When a user bypasses the CDN

9. Which protocol is commonly used by CDNs to serve web content quickly and efficiently?

a) FTP

b) HTTP/HTTPS

c) SMTP

d) SNMP

10. What does **content routing** in a CDN typically rely on to determine which edge server should deliver content?

a) The user's device type

b) Geographical location of the user

c) Server load

d) The file type being requested

11. A **load balancer** in a CDN architecture is used for:

a) Redirecting traffic to different edge servers based on their load

b) Increasing cache size

c) Monitoring TTL for content expiration

d) Authenticating user requests

12. Which mechanism in a CDN helps reduce the distance data travels between the user and the server?

   a) Dynamic caching

   b) Geolocation-based routing

   c) Reverse proxy

   d) Content encryption

13. What is the **origin server** responsible for in a CDN setup?

   a) Caching content for faster delivery

   b) Storing and providing the original content

   c) Managing user requests

   d) Load balancing traffic

14. In a CDN, what does the **geolocation of the user** determine?

   a) The content type requested

   b) Which edge server will deliver the content

   c) Whether the content will be cached

   d) The TTL for cached content

15. What happens when an edge server encounters a **cache miss**?

   a) It serves the content from its own cache

   b) It purges the cached content

   c) It requests the content from the origin server

   d) It redirects the user to another edge server

16. What is **load balancing** used for in a CDN?

   a) To distribute content across edge servers

   b) To allocate resources for content storage

   c) To direct user traffic to the least busy edge server

   d) To decide the TTL of cached files

17. What is the typical **cache expiration** strategy in a CDN?

   a) Caches never expire

   b) Files are cached indefinitely

   c) Content is cached based on TTL settings

   d) Content expires based on the user's device

18. What is the purpose of **dynamic content caching** in a CDN?

    a) To store images and static assets

    b) To speed up API responses and interactive content

    c) To reduce the size of files delivered

    d) To store encrypted data

19. What happens when a user requests content that has already been cached in an edge server?

    a) The request is forwarded to the origin server

    b) The content is delivered from the cache

    c) The content is re-cached

    d) The content is deleted from the cache

20. How does **DNS routing** work in a CDN?

    a) It caches DNS queries to speed up subsequent requests

    b) It directs users to the closest edge server based on their location

    c) It compresses DNS queries

    d) It prioritizes domain names over IP addresses

21. What does **content purging** refer to in CDN management?

    a) Removing expired content from cache

    b) Increasing cache size

    c) Encrypting cached data

    d) Creating new edge server locations

22. Which of the following is a **challenge** in CDN architecture?

    a) Reducing the TTL

    b) Managing cache size for dynamic content

    c) Encrypting data in transit

    d) Limiting edge server locations

23. In a CDN, **reverse proxy servers**:

    a) Authenticate users before delivering content

    b) Cache content closer to the user

    c) Route traffic to edge servers

    d) Load balance between the origin server and edge servers

24. How do CDNs handle **global scalability**?

    a) By using a single central server

    b) By distributing content across multiple edge servers worldwide

    c) By reducing the number of edge servers

    d) By caching content locally only

25. What is a **hybrid CDN**?

    a) A CDN that uses multiple origins

    b) A combination of traditional and cloud-based CDNs

    c) A CDN that relies only on local edge servers

    d) A CDN that does not cache content

26. Which component of a CDN is responsible for **request routing** to the closest edge server?

    a) Origin server

    b) Load balancer

    c) DNS server

    d) Content management system

27. Which **network protocol** is primarily used for data transfer between CDN servers and end-users?

    a) UDP

    b) HTTP/HTTPS

    c) FTP

    d) TCP

28. How do **CDN edge servers** improve the performance of **media streaming**?

    a) By reducing server load

    b) By caching video files closer to users

    c) By enabling adaptive bitrate streaming

    d) By reducing video compression

29. What role do **edge nodes** play in the architecture of **edge computing**?

    a) They process data at the point of generation to reduce latency

    b) They manage all content stored on the origin server

c) They directly monitor the security of all traffic

d) They are responsible for content encryption

30. What does the **caching strategy** of a CDN depend on?

    a) File size

    b) Content type (static vs. dynamic)

    c) User geolocation

    d) All of the above

31. What is a **content delivery network** primarily used for in a **global e-commerce site**?

    a) To deliver large files

    b) To speed up page load times and reduce latency

    c) To store data in a local database

    d) To handle user authentication

32. **CDN security** measures typically include:

    a) Data encryption and access control

    b) Caching sensitive data

    c) Serving content only from the origin server

    d) Reducing edge server locations

33. A **cache hit ratio** is defined as the percentage of:

    a) Requests served by the origin server

    b) Requests that do not require caching

    c) Requests served by the CDN cache rather than the origin server

    d) Requests that result in a cache miss

34. In a CDN, what is the purpose of **SSL/TLS encryption**?

    a) To encrypt user data at rest

    b) To ensure secure communication between users and the CDN servers

    c) To store encryption keys on the edge servers

    d) To manage content expiry

35. A **reverse proxy** in a CDN acts as:

    a) An intermediary that directs user requests to the origin server or edge server

    b) A system for managing user login data

c) A security feature that blocks malicious traffic

d) A tool for compressing files

36. Which of the following is the **main advantage** of using **dynamic content caching**?

    a) Reducing bandwidth usage

    b) Speeding up the delivery of content like APIs and user-generated data

    c) Storing large files on the edge servers

    d) Preventing security breaches

37. **Edge computing** is commonly integrated with CDNs to:

    a) Increase the security of cached content

    b) Enable local data processing closer to the end user

    c) Extend the TTL of content in the cache

    d) Encrypt all user data

38. What is **DNS caching** in the context of CDN?

    a) Storing DNS records at the edge servers to reduce DNS query time

    b) Storing content at the origin server

    c) Encrypting DNS queries between servers

    d) Reducing the number of DNS records

39. What happens to **stale content** in a CDN's cache when the TTL expires?

    a) It is purged from the cache

    b) It is automatically updated by the origin server

    c) It is transferred to another edge server

    d) It is kept until the user requests the content

40. What is the **primary function** of **CDN monitoring** tools?

    a) To encrypt content before delivery

    b) To track content delivery performance and troubleshoot issues

    c) To create new edge server locations

    d) To optimize image compression

41. **Real-time content delivery optimization** focuses on:

    a) Improving image quality

    b) Reducing latency and enhancing performance

c) Managing content expiration

d) Securing cached data

42. The **origin server** is primarily used to:

   a) Cache frequently requested content

   b) Store the original, unmodified version of content

   c) Handle the authentication of CDN users

   d) Redirect traffic to edge servers

43. **CDN traffic monitoring** tools can help identify:

   a) Popular content types

   b) Geographical traffic patterns

   c) Potential security threats

   d) All of the above

44. A **TTL mismatch** between edge servers and the origin server can lead to:

   a) Cache hits

   b) Stale content

   c) Increased latency

   d) Faster content delivery

45. What is the function of a **cache manager** in a CDN?

   a) To route user requests

   b) To monitor the TTL of cached content

   c) To handle user authentication

   d) To determine the best routing paths for content

46. What is **adaptive bitrate streaming** used for in a CDN?

   a) To improve the quality of static content

   b) To adjust video quality based on the user's bandwidth

   c) To compress audio files

   d) To ensure security of video content

47. A **reverse proxy** in CDN architecture is often responsible for:

   a) Encrypting data

   b) Caching content at the origin server

c) Distributing traffic among different edge servers

d) Compressing video streams

48. Which of the following is a **typical challenge** when caching **dynamic content** in a CDN?

a) Content change frequency

b) Large file size

c) Content expiration

d) Limited edge server locations

49. What does the **edge server** do when a user makes a request for content that is not available in its cache?

a) It delivers the content from the origin server

b) It redirects the request to another edge server

c) It serves an error message

d) It retrieves the content from another user's cache

50. How does **DNS load balancing** contribute to CDN performance?

a) It ensures content is cached properly

b) It routes traffic to the least-loaded edge server

c) It improves cache hit rates

d) It compresses DNS queries

51. **Content pre-fetching** in a CDN refers to:

a) Storing data in an edge server before it is requested by the user

b) Compressing content to speed up transfer

c) Encrypting content for security

d) Purging outdated content

52. A **CDN edge server** may include which of the following components for performance optimization?

a) Web acceleration technology

b) Content security protocols

c) Web application firewall (WAF)

d) All of the above

53. What does **content routing** rely on in order to provide the best user experience?

a) The file size

b) The user's geolocation

c) The browser type

d) The edge server's cache hit ratio

54. What is the key advantage of **edge caching** for **video content delivery** in a CDN?

    a) It reduces the video file size

    b) It increases video quality

    c) It minimizes buffering by serving the content from a nearby edge server

    d) It encrypts the video content

55. In a CDN architecture, **content routing algorithms** are responsible for:

    a) Deciding how content is stored in the cache

    b) Determining which edge server should deliver content based on the user's location

    c) Calculating the optimal TTL

    d) Encrypting the content

56. **Cloud-based CDNs** offer the advantage of:

    a) Hosting content solely on local servers

    b) Providing infinite scalability and global reach

    c) Delivering content only to specific countries

    d) Caching content locally on a single server

57. Which of the following strategies helps reduce **latency** in a CDN?

    a) Using a single large edge server

    b) Caching content at the origin server only

    c) Using multiple, geographically distributed edge servers

    d) Compressing all content

58. What is the main challenge of caching **dynamic content** in a CDN?

    a) Large content size

    b) Content is highly personalized and changes frequently

    c) Limited server storage

    d) Content encryption

59. What is a **content delivery node** (CDN node) typically responsible for?

    a) Load balancing

    b) Caching and delivering content

c) User authentication

d) DNS query management

60. Which of the following CDN technologies is used to improve **media streaming performance**?

a) Adaptive bitrate streaming

b) Static content compression

c) DNS query acceleration

d) Real-time analytics

61. How does **edge computing** benefit CDNs in terms of performance?

a) By processing data closer to the user, reducing latency

b) By compressing content in real-time

c) By offloading cache storage to the origin server

d) By filtering malicious traffic

62. A **cache refresh** occurs in a CDN when:

a) The content in the cache is outdated or stale

b) A cache hit occurs

c) A user requests content from a distant edge server

d) The DNS TTL expires

63. **Content pre-positioning** in a CDN is used to:

a) Ensure content is available before the user makes a request

b) Remove unwanted data from the cache

c) Increase the TTL of cached content

d) Protect content from DDoS attacks

64. In a CDN, **load balancing** typically helps with:

a) Redirecting traffic to different origin servers

b) Managing cache size

c) Distributing user requests across multiple edge servers

d) Caching dynamic content

65. What is the role of a **CDN proxy server**?

a) To cache user-specific content

b) To deliver content from the origin server directly

c) To act as an intermediary between the user and the edge server

d) To monitor user behavior

66. **Geolocation-based routing** in a CDN is designed to:

   a) Serve content from the server with the lowest cost

   b) Reduce the time to find content on the origin server

   c) Direct user requests to the nearest edge server for faster content delivery

   d) Compress content during transmission

67. What type of content is most commonly **cached** in a CDN?

   a) Static content such as images, CSS, and JavaScript

   b) Dynamic content such as user profiles and comments

   c) Content that requires frequent updates

   d) Large video files

68. **CDN security features** typically include:

   a) SSL/TLS encryption

   b) DDoS protection

   c) Web application firewall (WAF)

   d) All of the above

69. **SSL termination** in a CDN refers to:

   a) Encrypting all content delivered to the user

   b) Decrypting SSL-encrypted traffic at the edge server to reduce load on the origin server

   c) Encrypting content on the origin server

   d) Redirecting user traffic through a secure proxy

70. **Content delivery acceleration** in a CDN aims to:

   a) Speed up the encryption process

   b) Minimize the time it takes to deliver content to users

   c) Increase cache hit ratios

   d) Encrypt all user data

71. How do **CDNs optimize the delivery of APIs**?

   a) By caching API responses at edge servers

   b) By reducing the time to query APIs

c) By encrypting API keys

d) By using different API formats

72. What is **content invalidation** in a CDN?

    a) The process of ensuring that cached content is always valid

    b) The process of removing outdated or incorrect content from the cache

    c) The process of renewing the TTL for cached files

    d) The process of encrypting content during transmission

73. Which type of **content** is best suited for **edge caching**?

    a) Dynamic content that changes frequently

    b) Static content such as images and videos

    c) Personalized content for individual users

    d) Real-time data streams

74. What does a **Content Delivery Network (CDN)** optimize for when serving media content?

    a) File compression

    b) Geographic content delivery

    c) User authentication

    d) Bandwidth usage

75. The **primary purpose of DNS-based CDN routing** is to:

    a) Securely store content at the edge servers

    b) Direct user requests to the appropriate edge server based on location

    c) Compress DNS queries

    d) Cache DNS records at the origin server

76. A **web application firewall (WAF)** integrated with a CDN is used to:

    a) Protect content from unauthorized access

    b) Cache data at the origin server

    c) Accelerate content delivery

    d) Compress large video files

77. Which of the following would **most benefit** from the use of a CDN?

    a) A small local blog

    b) A global e-commerce platform

c) A single-page website

d) A website with limited global traffic

78. Which of the following is a **real-time content delivery** strategy used by CDNs?

    a) Pre-fetching content based on usage patterns

    b) Dynamic content caching

    c) Adaptive bitrate streaming

    d) All of the above

79. What does **cache evicting** mean in a CDN?

    a) Removing expired content from cache

    b) Increasing the TTL of cached files

    c) Storing new content in the origin server

    d) Sending content to a different edge server

80. **API acceleration** by a CDN primarily focuses on:

    a) Compressing API responses

    b) Reducing the time it takes to serve API data

    c) Encrypting API keys

    d) Storing user credentials

81. Which of the following strategies can help **CDNs** handle **high traffic volumes**?

    a) Deploying additional edge servers

    b) Using only origin servers

    c) Compressing content heavily

    d) Reducing DNS query size

82. The use of **secure edge servers** in a CDN helps mitigate:

    a) Content piracy

    b) Malware and DDoS attacks

    c) Long load times

    d) Cache expiry

83. What type of **CDN monitoring** tool provides insights into **user behavior and traffic patterns**?

    a) Performance monitoring tools

    b) Security analysis tools

c) Real-time analytics tools

d) All of the above

84. The **longer the TTL**, the:

a) Faster the content delivery

b) Longer the cached content stays valid in the edge server

c) More frequent the content updates

d) Lower the security

85. Which of the following is an important factor in deciding **TTL settings** for cached content?

a) Content type (static or dynamic)

b) Content security requirements

c) Content update frequency

d) All of the above

86. **CDN peering** refers to:

a) The practice of connecting multiple CDNs for content sharing

b) The sharing of edge servers across regions

c) The distribution of content based on content type

d) The process of transferring user data

87. **Real-time analytics** in a CDN environment can help with:

a) Tracking cache hit and miss rates

b) Identifying performance bottlenecks

c) Monitoring user behavior and traffic

d) All of the above

88. What is the **main goal** of **geographically distributed edge servers** in a CDN?

a) To store data for faster access

b) To provide users with content from the closest possible server

c) To encrypt data during transfer

d) To reduce traffic loads on origin servers

89. **High availability** in a CDN is achieved by:

a) Increasing the number of edge servers globally

b) Using a single origin server

c) Disabling caching mechanisms

d) Storing all content in the origin server

90. Which factor affects **cache hit ratio** in a CDN?

a) Content popularity

b) TTL settings

c) Content type (static vs. dynamic)

d) All of the above

91. **DDoS mitigation** by a CDN often includes:

a) Caching all content

b) Rate-limiting and traffic filtering

c) Using multiple origin servers

d) Encrypting all traffic

92. Which of the following strategies can be used to improve **content delivery speed** in a CDN?

a) Reducing file size through compression

b) Using edge caching and load balancing

c) Serving content based on geolocation

d) All of the above

93. What does a **CDN origin shield** do?

a) Protects content from unauthorized access

b) Shields the origin server from high traffic loads by serving requests from edge servers

c) Encrypts all data delivered by the CDN

d) Compresses content

94. **Cache invalidation** in a CDN can be triggered by:

a) TTL expiration

b) Manual purging

c) Content updates from the origin server

d) All of the above

95. Which of the following technologies does a CDN use to optimize **media content delivery**?

a) Adaptive bitrate streaming

b) Content encryption

c) Dynamic content caching

d) Traffic shaping

96. What is a key benefit of **multi-CDN strategies**?

    a) Improved performance through redundancy

    b) Lower content delivery costs

    c) Simpler architecture

    d) Reduced security risks

97. **Global load balancing** in a CDN helps ensure:

    a) High-speed delivery of content worldwide

    b) All content is cached

    c) Content is encrypted

    d) Single point of access for all users

98. **Caching strategies** used in a CDN depend on:

    a) Content type

    b) User preferences

    c) Security requirements

    d) All of the above

99. The **most common caching strategy** for **static content** is:

    a) Cache for a long time based on TTL

    b) Never cache

    c) Cache based on user location

    d) Cache dynamically

100.   **Edge nodes** in a CDN primarily aim to:

    a) Process content updates

    b) Deliver content with low latency

    c) Store content permanently

    d) Monitor network traffic

CDN Performance and Optimization:

1. Which of the following is the most common cause of **latency** in CDN content delivery?

A) Distance between the user and the edge server

B) The size of the file being delivered

C) The format of the content

D) The origin server's hardware capacity

2. What is the primary advantage of **caching** in a CDN?

A) It reduces the amount of content on the origin server

B) It ensures data security by encrypting files

C) It speeds up the delivery of content to users by storing copies closer to them

D) It increases the cost of content delivery

3. Time to Live (TTL) in CDN caching defines:

A) The maximum time a cached content will be stored on edge servers

B) The total time content spends on the origin server

C) How often the content should be encrypted

D) The time it takes for data to reach the user from the origin server

4. In a CDN, **cache hits** are:

A) When content is not available in the cache and must be retrieved from the origin server

B) When content is served from the CDN cache instead of the origin server

C) When content is purged from the cache

D) When content is modified and stored in the cache

5. Cache misses in a CDN occur when:

A) Content is served from the edge server cache

B) The content is too large for the cache

C) The requested content is not in the cache and must be fetched from the origin

D) The cache is full and must purge older data

6. What is **adaptive bitrate streaming** used for in CDN optimization?

A) To adjust video quality based on the viewer's bandwidth

B) To compress video files for faster delivery

C) To store video content in multiple formats

D) To encrypt video content during delivery

7. Pre-fetching content in a CDN involves:

A) Compressing content before storing it in the cache

B) Storing content at the edge server before it is requested

C) Removing old content from the cache

D) Encrypting content before it is cached

8. Content purging in a CDN refers to:

A) Updating content stored in the cache

B) Removing outdated or stale content from the cache

C) Compressing content before caching

D) Encrypting content stored at the origin

9. What is the purpose of **dynamic content caching** in a CDN?

A) To store content that changes frequently for faster delivery

B) To reduce the storage size of cached content

C) To deliver personalized content based on the user

D) To encrypt dynamic content

10. Edge caching primarily reduces the impact of:

A) High traffic volumes on the origin server

B) Large file sizes

C) Content security risks

D) User privacy issues

11. The **TTL setting** for cached content is important because it determines:

A) The cost of content delivery

B) How long the content remains valid in the cache

C) The encryption level of the content

D) The maximum storage limit for cached content

12. To optimize CDN performance, **content delivery speed** is improved by:

A) Reducing the TTL for all cached content

B) Increasing the number of origin servers

C) Using geographically distributed edge servers

D) Encrypting all content before delivery

13. Which of the following **caching strategies** would be most appropriate for **static content**?

A) Cache for a long duration based on TTL

B) Never cache static content

C) Cache dynamically based on user requests

D) Only cache static content in certain regions

14. Geolocation-based routing in a CDN improves performance by:

A) Routing traffic to the server with the least load

B) Sending content to the nearest edge server based on user location

C) Reducing DNS query time

D) Encrypting all data during delivery

15. Content compression in a CDN helps to:

A) Reduce the file size and accelerate delivery

B) Increase the quality of the content

C) Secure content from unauthorized access

D) Store content more efficiently on the origin server

16. In a CDN, **load balancing** ensures that:

A) All edge servers handle equal traffic

B) Traffic is redirected to the origin server

C) The cache hit ratio is maximized

D) Content is served from the closest edge server

17. Real-time optimization in a CDN refers to:

A) Dynamically adjusting caching strategies based on current traffic

B) Preloading content before it is requested

C) Compressing content in real-time

D) Encrypting content during transmission

18. Edge servers are beneficial for CDN performance because they:

A) Store content at the origin server

B) Serve content from locations closer to the user, reducing latency

C) Encrypt content for enhanced security

D) Perform complex computational tasks

19. Cache eviction in a CDN occurs when:

A) New content replaces outdated content in the cache

B) Cached content is manually removed

C) A user requests content that is not in the cache

D) The TTL for cached content expires

20. The **use of multiple CDNs** (multi-CDN strategy) helps improve performance by:

A) Reducing the time it takes to find content on the origin server

B) Providing redundancy and avoiding single points of failure

C) Increasing the cache size at edge servers

D) Encrypting all traffic

21. A **content delivery node** (CDN node) is responsible for:

A) Serving requests from the origin server

B) Caching and delivering content from the edge

C) Storing content permanently

D) Monitoring traffic across the CDN

22. CDN traffic shaping involves:

A) Compressing data to improve load times

B) Managing the flow of traffic based on current network conditions

C) Encrypting data for secure delivery

D) Increasing the TTL of cached content

23. The goal of **load balancing** in CDN optimization is to:

A) Ensure that content is always served from the origin server

B) Spread user requests across multiple edge servers to prevent overload

C) Prioritize traffic from certain users

D) Reduce the size of the content delivered

24. Content pre-positioning in a CDN can help optimize performance by:

A) Storing content closer to users before they request it

B) Compressing content during delivery

C) Encrypting content during transfer

D) Removing old content from the cache

25. DNS-based routing in a CDN improves performance by:

A) Compressing DNS requests to reduce latency

B) Directing users to the nearest available edge server

C) Ensuring that all DNS requests are encrypted

D) Storing DNS queries in the cache

26. To minimize **latency** when delivering **video content**, CDNs often use:

A) Adaptive bitrate streaming

B) File compression

C) Data encryption

D) Multi-CDN strategies

27. Which of the following is a **key benefit** of **edge caching** for **static content**?

A) Faster content delivery by storing it closer to the user

B) Increased security by encrypting content

C) Dynamic adjustment of content based on user preferences

D) Larger storage capacity at the origin server

28. Real-time analytics in CDN performance monitoring is used to:

A) Track the performance of edge servers

B) Understand user behavior

C) Optimize cache hit rates

D) All of the above

29. The primary challenge of **caching dynamic content** in a CDN is:

A) Frequent changes in content

B) Large file sizes

C) User authentication requirements

D) Difficulty in compressing dynamic content

30. The **use of edge servers** in a CDN improves delivery by:

A) Compressing all content before delivery

B) Storing content at the origin server

C) Reducing the distance content must travel to reach the user

D) Ensuring content is encrypted

31. Reducing cache misses in a CDN improves:

A) User security

B) Cache hit ratios

C) Content compression rates

D) Video quality

32. Cache hit ratios in a CDN can be improved by:

A) Increasing the TTL for static content

B) Using only a single edge server

C) Reducing the number of edge servers

D) Serving content only from the origin server

33. Compression techniques in a CDN reduce content size by:

A) Minimizing the file format used

B) Removing non-essential content

C) Encoding the content in a more efficient format

D) Increasing the TTL of cached content

34. What is the primary function of **origin shield** in CDN optimization?

A) To protect the origin server from high traffic volumes by handling requests at the edge

B) To encrypt all content before it is cached

C) To compress content during delivery

D) To increase the TTL of cached content

35. DDoS attacks can be mitigated by CDNs using:

A) Rate-limiting and filtering suspicious traffic

B) Storing all traffic on origin servers

C) Caching content at the origin server

D) Increasing the cache hit rate

36. Edge caching helps optimize **video streaming** by:

A) Storing multiple versions of video content at the edge

B) Reducing the size of video files during delivery

C) Ensuring secure delivery of video files

D) Limiting the bitrate of video content

37. Load balancing between CDNs helps:

A) Optimize content delivery across regions

B) Increase storage at the origin server

C) Encrypt content more effectively

D) Ensure all content is cached in all regions

38. Geo-replication in a CDN improves performance by:

A) Storing multiple copies of content at edge servers in different geographic regions

B) Encrypting all content at the origin server

C) Limiting the amount of content cached

D) Disabling caching for sensitive data

39. Traffic management in CDNs aims to:

A) Control the flow of content from the origin server to the user

B) Optimize the number of edge servers

C) Ensure content is cached for long periods

D) Prioritize requests from specific users

40. The goal of **pre-fetching content** in a CDN is to:

A) Reduce the time it takes for users to receive content

B) Increase security by storing encrypted copies

C) Store large amounts of content on the origin server

D) Compress files before storing them in the cache

41. Edge computing in the context of a CDN refers to:

A) Performing computation tasks closer to the user to reduce latency

B) Storing all content at the origin server

C) Encrypting data at the origin server

D) Compressing content before delivery

42. CDN performance monitoring involves tracking:

A) Cache hit/miss rates

B) Content delivery speed

C) Server load and health

D) All of the above

43. To optimize **content delivery** for **mobile users**, CDNs typically:

A) Use lower TTL settings

B) Compress files more aggressively

C) Use adaptive bitrate streaming

D) Use edge servers only in urban areas

44. Caching dynamic content at the edge is challenging because:

A) It changes frequently

B) It is larger than static content

C) It requires secure storage

D) It is encrypted before delivery

45. What is the purpose of **DNS-level routing** in CDN performance optimization?

A) To ensure faster DNS resolution by caching queries

B) To direct user requests to the most efficient edge server

C) To filter out malicious traffic

D) To prioritize high-value content

46. Cache eviction in CDN refers to:

A) The process of deleting outdated content from the cache

B) Compressing content before caching

C) Encrypting content before it is stored

D) Retrieving content from the origin server

47. Edge nodes in a CDN aim to:

A) Increase security

B) Serve content with lower latency

C) Compress data

D) Perform computational tasks

48. Caching of media content (e.g., videos) in a CDN can be optimized by:

A) Reducing the quality of the content

B) Using adaptive bitrate streaming

C) Encrypting the content before delivery

D) Compressing the content before caching

49. The **main benefit** of **multi-CDN strategies** is:

A) Increased redundancy and reliability

B) Reduced overall cache hit rates

C) Higher content delivery costs

D) Simplified infrastructure management

50. Content prepositioning helps to:

A) Store content before users request it

B) Ensure that content is encrypted

C) Reduce content size

D) Automatically purge content from the cache

51. The **primary benefit of CDN caching** is:

A) Improved content delivery speed by serving content from the closest edge server

B) Increased cost due to additional storage requirements

C) Reduced redundancy in content delivery

D) Ensured content encryption

52. Adaptive bitrate streaming improves CDN performance by:

A) Reducing the number of edge servers required

B) Dynamically adjusting video quality to fit the user's available bandwidth

C) Compressing content for faster delivery

D) Encrypting media files

53. **What is the impact of a low **cache hit ratio** on CDN performance?

A) Increased traffic to the origin server, leading to higher latency

B) Reduced security

C) Faster content delivery to users

D) Improved cache performance

54. The **purpose of content pre-fetching** in CDN is to:

A) Minimize latency by proactively storing frequently requested content on edge servers

B) Encrypt content to ensure privacy

C) Compress content to save bandwidth

D) Cache content for a longer TTL

55. A **dynamic content delivery strategy** for CDNs focuses on:

A) Caching static files only

B) Optimizing the delivery of personalized, frequently changing content

C) Increasing cache TTL for all content

D) Compressing all dynamic content for storage

56. Cache consistency in CDN systems is maintained by:

A) Having edge servers periodically refresh their cached content from the origin server

B) Encrypting all content

C) Using multiple origin servers

D) Compressing content

57. The **main reason for using a CDN** in delivering media content is:

A) To increase the security of the content

B) To reduce the time it takes for content to reach the user by serving it from the nearest edge server

C) To encrypt all media content during delivery

D) To store all media content at the origin server

58. Geo-blocking in a CDN involves:

A) Limiting access to content based on the user's geographical location

B) Storing content only in certain regions

C) Encrypting content for specific regions

D) Reducing the number of edge servers

59. Cache purging is required in a CDN when:

A) Content is updated on the origin server and needs to be refreshed at the edge servers

B) The TTL for content expires

C) Content becomes outdated or irrelevant

D) All of the above

60. Edge server replication in a CDN helps with:

A) Distributing content closer to users

B) Increasing the number of origin servers

C) Improving security through encryption

D) Reducing the amount of content stored on edge servers

61. Real-time CDN analytics provide insights on:

A) Cache hit/miss rates, traffic patterns, and user behavior

B) Only cache hit ratios

C) The content's size and format

D) The time taken to process DNS queries

**62. **What is the role of **content delivery networks in mobile optimization?

A) To compress mobile content to fit smaller screens

B) To reduce the time it takes to deliver content to mobile devices

C) To ensure mobile-specific content is encrypted

D) To store content on mobile devices for offline use

63. Latency in CDN performance is defined as:

A) The amount of time it takes to encrypt content

B) The time it takes for data to travel from the origin server to the user

C) The time spent storing content in the cache

D) The time it takes to purge content from the cache

64. CDN edge nodes can improve performance by:

A) Hosting the content at the origin server

B) Storing content closer to the user, reducing the load on the origin server

C) Encrypting all content

D) Handling all traffic without load balancing

65. Which of the following factors **affects content caching performance** in a CDN?

A) Content type (static or dynamic)

B) Cache TTL settings

C) Edge server distribution

D) All of the above

66. A **high cache hit ratio** in a CDN leads to:

A) Lower latency and faster content delivery

B) Increased traffic to the origin server

C) More frequent content purging

D) Higher content delivery costs

67. Cache busting refers to:

A) Using unique URLs for updated content to force the CDN to retrieve the latest version

B) Increasing the TTL for all cached content

C) Encrypting content to prevent unauthorized access

D) Compressing content for faster delivery

68. Edge caching can improve CDN performance by:

A) Decreasing the load on the origin server

B) Reducing content delivery time by storing copies closer to users

C) Enhancing security through encryption

D) A and B

69. Performance bottlenecks in a CDN can be caused by:

A) Slow origin server response times

B) Inadequate edge server locations

C) High traffic volumes during peak hours

D) All of the above

70. **What is the role of **load balancing** in a CDN system?

A) To evenly distribute traffic across multiple edge servers

B) To ensure that all traffic is routed through a single server

C) To prioritize specific types of traffic for faster delivery

D) To compress data during delivery

71. Multi-CDN strategies can improve performance by:

A) Increasing redundancy and reliability through the use of different CDN providers

B) Reducing the TTL for all content

C) Compressing content across all CDNs

D) Increasing security by using multiple encryption methods

72. **What does CDN optimization for mobile devices generally focus on?**

A) Reducing content size and increasing cache TTL

B) Delivering smaller, optimized versions of content for mobile screens

C) Ensuring that content is encrypted

D) Storing content on mobile devices for offline access

73. Content delivery speed can be improved in a CDN by:

A) Using edge servers that are geographically closer to the user

B) Reducing the size of the content

C) Compressing the content

D) All of the above

74. CDN traffic analysis helps to:

A) Understand patterns in content requests and optimize cache performance

B) Improve content security

C) Increase the storage capacity of the origin server

D) Identify malicious traffic only

75. CDN caching rules should be defined based on:

A) The frequency of content updates

B) Content type (static or dynamic)

C) Security requirements

D) All of the above

76. Reducing latency in a CDN primarily involves:

A) Storing content on origin servers

B) Using content delivery nodes that are closer to users

C) Encrypting all content before delivery

D) Compressing content during transmission

77. Content pre-positioning is helpful for optimizing:

A) Static content delivery by storing content in advance at edge servers

B) Dynamic content by serving it from the origin server

C) Encrypted content for secure delivery

D) Content that does not change frequently

78. A **high-quality CDN provider** should offer:

A) Global coverage with edge servers in various regions

B) Advanced security features like DDoS protection

C) Real-time analytics and performance monitoring tools

D) All of the above

79. Load balancing between multiple edge servers helps optimize:

A) The user experience by reducing wait times

B) Content encryption

C) The storage space of origin servers

D) The complexity of DNS routing

80. **What is a key **difference between static and dynamic content caching** in CDNs?

A) Static content rarely changes, so it can be cached for longer periods, while dynamic content requires more frequent updates in the cache

B) Dynamic content is always cached at the edge, while static content is only cached at the origin server

C) Static content is smaller in size and easier to cache

D) Dynamic content is encrypted by default

81. Reducing cache misses in a CDN can be achieved by:

A) Using edge servers strategically to increase cache hit ratios

B) Decreasing the TTL for all content

C) Storing dynamic content exclusively on the origin server

D) Encrypting all content

82. A **low cache hit ratio** in a CDN is likely caused by:

A) Using too many edge servers

B) A large proportion of dynamic content that cannot be cached efficiently

C) Too high a TTL value for content

D) Increased use of pre-fetched content

83. CDN performance optimization for **video streaming** involves:

A) Adaptive bitrate streaming and edge caching of video content

B) Reducing video file size by increasing compression

C) Encrypting all video content

D) None of the above

84. The **primary objective** of **multi-CDN strategies** is:

A) To improve reliability and reduce risks associated with reliance on a single CDN provider

B) To ensure content is cached at every edge server

C) To compress content for faster delivery

D) To encrypt content at all stages of delivery

85. **What is the role of **DNS-based routing** in CDN optimization?

A) To improve content delivery speed by directing requests to the nearest edge server

B) To ensure all content is encrypted

C) To reduce traffic to the origin server by caching requests

D) To perform load balancing

86. Content delivery optimization in CDNs can be enhanced by:

A) Using real-time traffic data to adjust caching rules dynamically

B) Compressing all content before delivery

C) Reducing the number of edge servers

D) Ignoring geolocation for content routing

87. What is the main challenge when caching **dynamic content** in a CDN?

A) Frequent changes to the content that require frequent cache updates

B) Larger file sizes

C) Content encryption

D) User-specific content

88. Edge computing in the context of CDN optimization is used for:

A) Reducing the need to send data back to the origin server for computation

B) Encrypting content before transmission

C) Caching data on mobile devices

D) Reducing server costs by eliminating edge nodes

89. **How do **real-time CDN optimizations** enhance performance?

A) By dynamically adjusting caching, content routing, and traffic management based on current network conditions

B) By reducing the number of edge servers

C) By only caching static content

D) By encrypting all traffic

90. Traffic monitoring in a CDN helps improve performance by:

A) Understanding user behavior and optimizing cache delivery

B) Encrypting sensitive data

C) Reducing the number of edge servers used

D) Reducing the size of content delivered

91. **Why is **content pre-positioning** useful for CDNs?

A) It helps serve content faster by storing popular content on edge servers in advance

B) It allows content to be compressed

C) It reduces the number of edge servers needed

D) It increases the TTL of cached content

92. Cache purging in a CDN is most commonly used to:

A) Update stale or outdated content in the cache

B) Compress content before storage

C) Improve security by encrypting content

D) Remove duplicate content

93. Multi-CDN deployment provides which of the following benefits?

A) Increased performance and redundancy

B) Higher content delivery costs

C) More centralized content management

D) Reduced caching capabilities

94. **How does **traffic routing** in CDNs contribute to optimization?

A) By directing users to the fastest and closest edge server based on their geographic location

B) By using only one edge server

C) By encrypting content

D) By reducing the amount of content cached

95. What type of content benefits the most from **CDN caching**?

A) Static content such as images, scripts, and videos

B) Highly personalized content

C) Secure, encrypted content

D) Dynamic content

96. What is the main challenge in **optimizing media streaming** over CDNs?

A) Ensuring adaptive bitrate streaming and efficient caching

B) Encrypting content

C) Increasing the size of content

D) Managing DNS queries

97. A CDN edge server is best suited for:

A) Serving content quickly from geographically distributed locations

B) Hosting all content on the origin server

C) Encrypting all content

D) Compressing content at the origin

98. Cache hit ratios can be improved by:

A) Reducing the TTL of content

B) Storing frequently accessed content at edge nodes

C) Increasing the number of edge servers

D) A and B

99. Real-time optimization techniques in a CDN are primarily focused on:

A) Adjusting delivery strategies based on network conditions and traffic volume

B) Storing content at the origin server

C) Encrypting content during transfer

D) Compressing content before storage

100. Using multiple CDN providers helps optimize:

A) Redundancy and reliability of content delivery

B) Traffic to origin servers

C) Content encryption

D) Content size

Advanced CDN Techniques

1. What is **Edge Computing** in the context of CDNs?

A) Storing data on cloud servers

B) Processing data closer to the user to reduce latency

C) Increasing the security of content

D) Encrypting data at the origin server

2. Which of the following is a key advantage of using **Serverless architecture** in a CDN?

A) Reduced need for edge nodes

B) Scalability and flexibility in handling traffic

C) Increased content caching

D) Reduced security risks

3. **What is the purpose of **origin shield** in CDN architecture?

A) To serve content faster by storing more copies of it

B) To increase the cache hit rate by caching content closer to the user

C) To act as an additional layer of caching that protects the origin server

D) To enforce security protocols for sensitive data

4. Real-time optimization in a CDN refers to:

A) Compressing content during transmission

B) Dynamically adjusting delivery based on network conditions and demand

C) Storing content permanently in caches

D) Encrypting content before delivery

5. Which CDN technique helps minimize the **impact of DDoS attacks**?

A) Rate-limiting and filtering malicious traffic

B) Using stronger encryption

C) Increasing TTL for all content

D) Caching content at multiple edge servers

6. DNS-level routing in CDNs is primarily used to:

A) Compress content

B) Route requests to the nearest edge server

C) Improve content encryption

D) Increase the TTL of cached content

7. Content delivery latency can be reduced by:

A) Using a single origin server

B) Optimizing edge server placement and routing

C) Storing only static content

D) Disabling SSL encryption

8. Which of the following is the **key advantage of multi-CDN** strategies?

A) Reduced reliance on a single CDN provider

B) Higher content delivery costs

C) Increased complexity in content management

D) Simplified content security

9. Edge computing integration in CDNs can:

A) Store more content in origin servers

B) Improve data processing by handling computation closer to the user

C) Encrypt content for security

D) Reduce the number of CDN providers used

10. Serverless CDN optimizations help reduce:

A) Content delivery speed

B) Operational complexity and server management

C) Latency at the origin server

D) The need for content purging

11. Advanced caching strategies in CDNs include:

A) Cache purging on every update

B) Setting shorter TTL for all content

C) Cache segmentation based on content type and region

D) Storing dynamic content only

12. Which of the following is true about **dynamic content caching**?

A) It is always cached at the origin server

B) It must be cached for long TTL to avoid frequent cache misses

C) It can be cached at edge servers but requires more complex rules

D) It cannot be cached by CDNs

13. What is the role of **load balancing** in CDN performance optimization?

A) To ensure content is encrypted

B) To evenly distribute traffic across edge servers

C) To store content on origin servers

D) To cache content more efficiently

14. Edge caching in CDNs primarily benefits:

A) Large files that rarely change

B) Dynamic content that is highly personalized

C) Frequent updates to content

D) Low-latency delivery of content to users

15. The purpose of **pre-fetching content** in CDN systems is to:

A) Store content in advance to ensure quick delivery when requested

B) Compress content for faster transfer

C) Encrypt content before caching

D) Cache all content for an extended TTL

16. Global load balancing across multiple CDN providers helps with:

A) Reducing server costs

B) Improving fault tolerance and service reliability

C) Compressing traffic

D) Encrypting traffic between servers

17. Content pre-positioning in CDN architecture refers to:

A) Storing content closer to users in advance of actual requests

B) Dynamically optimizing the size of content

C) Compressing content for faster delivery

D) Disabling caching for sensitive content

18. Edge node replication enhances CDN performance by:

A) Creating redundant copies of content in multiple geographic locations

B) Reducing content encryption

C) Minimizing the need for origin server requests

D) Ensuring content is cached at every edge node

19. What role does **real-time traffic analytics** play in CDN optimization?

A) It helps in the dynamic adjustment of caching rules and routing strategies

B) It is used to encrypt traffic to ensure privacy

C) It compresses traffic before transmission

D) It focuses only on monitoring traffic volume

20. Which technique is used to optimize **video content delivery** in a CDN?

A) Reducing video size for faster streaming

B) Adaptive bitrate streaming

C) Using shorter TTL for video content

D) Encrypting video files before delivery

21. How do CDNs use **machine learning** for performance optimization?

A) To automatically cache content based on demand patterns

B) To store content more efficiently on origin servers

C) To compress all content dynamically

D) To perform traffic analysis for security

22. What is the purpose of **edge caching** in video streaming?

A) To store large video files on origin servers

B) To ensure low-latency delivery and high-quality playback

C) To compress video files before caching

D) To enforce stricter security protocols

23. Which **load balancing method** is best suited for handling **high traffic spikes**?

A) Round-robin load balancing

B) DNS-based routing

C) Geographic-based load balancing

D) Randomized load balancing

24. What is **cache eviction**?

A) Removing outdated or irrelevant content from the cache to make room for fresh content

B) Compressing content to reduce storage space

C) Encrypting content before storing it in the cache

D) Dividing content into smaller segments for faster delivery

25. What is the benefit of **adaptive caching** strategies in CDNs?

A) Faster cache misses

B) Reduced latency by adapting to content access patterns

C) Increased security through content encryption

D) Simplified DNS routing

26. Which of the following is a benefit of **multi-region** caching in CDNs?

A) Increased load on origin servers

B) Reduced content delivery latency for global users

C) More frequent cache purging

D) Higher costs for storage

27. CDN traffic management aims to:

A) Distribute traffic evenly across multiple edge servers

B) Prioritize requests from users in specific regions

C) Direct all requests to the origin server

D) Encrypt traffic to prevent data breaches

28. What is the main challenge in **caching dynamic content**?

A) It changes frequently and may require updates in real-time

B) It is large and cannot be stored at edge servers

C) It cannot be encrypted

D) It is more susceptible to DDoS attacks

29. What is **cache segmentation** in advanced CDN configurations?

A) Dividing content into categories for more efficient caching

B) Compressing cached content into smaller chunks

C) Storing content only on the origin server

D) Encrypting content before caching

30. CDN performance tuning often involves:

A) Adjusting TTLs, cache rules, and load balancing strategies

B) Encrypting all content

C) Storing all content on the origin server

D) Disabling cache eviction

31. What is **edge-to-origin optimization** in a CDN?

A) Caching content at the edge for faster delivery

B) Reducing the amount of traffic between edge servers and the origin

C) Increasing the TTL of cached content

D) Compressing all traffic to reduce bandwidth usage

32. What is the benefit of using **multiple CDN providers** in an advanced strategy?

A) Reduced reliance on a single CDN provider for better redundancy

B) Higher content delivery costs

C) Increased complexity in managing caches

D) Reduced content security risks

33. What is the role of **edge servers** in CDN performance optimization?

A) To handle computation tasks

B) To deliver content quickly to users by being geographically close

C) To store all content in the cache

D) To perform encryption of content

34. Real-time content optimization in CDNs helps in:

A) Adjusting content delivery based on current traffic and network conditions

B) Increasing the amount of content cached

C) Encrypting all content during delivery

D) Compressing content for storage

35. Which of the following techniques is used to **reduce **origin server load** in CDNs?

A) Using **edge caching** for static content

B) Increasing TTL for all cached content

C) Storing dynamic content on the origin server

D) Using DNS-level routing for all requests

36. What does **DNS-level load balancing** help achieve in CDNs?

A) Redirecting user requests to the most efficient edge server

B) Compressing content before transmission

C) Encrypting all traffic

D) Storing dynamic content more efficiently

37. Which of the following technologies helps CDNs deliver **secure content** efficiently?

A) Edge encryption

B) Real-time traffic monitoring

C) Load balancing

D) Geolocation-based routing

38. What is the primary benefit of **using HTTP/2** in a CDN?

A) Improved content compression

B) Faster content delivery due to multiplexing and header compression

C) Enhanced security through encryption

D) Reduced origin server load

39. How does **WebAssembly** impact CDN performance optimization?

A) It allows content to be processed at the edge, reducing latency

B) It compresses all content before delivery

C) It increases content encryption security

D) It ensures all content is cached globally

40. Which caching technique improves content delivery by caching **user-specific content**?

A) Cache segmentation

B) Edge purging

C) Dynamic content caching

D) Cache bypassing

41. What is **content delivery pre-fetching**?

A) Predicting and loading content into cache before it is requested

B) Compressing content for delivery

C) Encrypting content before it is stored

D) Caching content only at the origin server

42. How does **cache hit ratio** impact CDN performance?

A) A higher cache hit ratio leads to faster content delivery and reduced load on origin servers

B) A higher cache hit ratio leads to slower content delivery

C) Cache hit ratio does not affect performance

D) A higher cache hit ratio reduces the security of content

43. In a multi-CDN setup, the role of **traffic steering** is to:

A) Dynamically route requests to the best-performing CDN provider based on real-time data

B) Store all content on a single CDN provider's edge servers

C) Cache content across multiple regions without considering performance

D) Compress traffic during routing to save bandwidth

44. What is **geo-aware caching** in a CDN?

A) Caching content closer to the user based on their geographical location

B) Encrypting content according to the user's region

C) Storing content based on the device type

D) Routing all traffic through a single data center

45. What is **real-time traffic analysis** used for in CDN optimization?

A) To adjust delivery strategies based on current traffic, device, and network conditions

B) To increase TTL for all cached content

C) To compress and encrypt all traffic before transmission

D) To optimize DNS routing based on historical data

46. Edge compute functions in CDNs help to:

A) Offload processing tasks closer to the user and reduce latency

B) Increase storage requirements for cached content

C) Improve DNS routing performance

D) Prevent content encryption

47. What is the benefit of **using TLS termination** at the edge in CDNs?

A) Offloading SSL/TLS encryption tasks to edge servers to reduce load on the origin server

B) Caching content more efficiently at the edge

C) Compressing content before encryption

D) Encrypting all content at the origin server

48. Which of the following best describes **cache purging**?

A) Deleting outdated or stale content from caches to allow fresh content to be stored

B) Compressing content before storing it in the cache

C) Encrypting content in the cache for security purposes

D) Storing only static content in the cache

49. What does **cache segmentation** help achieve in advanced CDN techniques?

A) It helps store content in different caches based on usage patterns and content types

B) It compresses content for faster delivery

C) It encrypts content during storage

D) It limits the number of edge servers used for caching

50. Why would a CDN use **real-time DNS routing**?

A) To direct users to the best-performing edge server based on geographic location and network conditions

B) To encrypt all content

C) To cache content at origin servers

D) To prevent cache evictions

51. What is **dynamic content caching** in CDNs?

A) Caching content that changes frequently, such as user-specific data, with a short TTL

B) Caching content at the origin server for long durations

C) Compressing content to reduce cache size

D) Storing only static content in the cache

52. Why is **multi-layer caching** important in a CDN setup?

A) To improve content delivery performance by caching content at various layers of the network

B) To reduce the need for load balancing

C) To prevent the caching of sensitive data

D) To increase the TTL of cached content

53. Which optimization technique is commonly used to reduce **origin server load** in CDNs?

A) Using edge caching for static content

B) Storing dynamic content exclusively at the origin

C) Increasing the TTL for all content

D) Compressing content at the origin server

54. What is **edge logic** in a CDN context?

A) Implementing logic at the edge servers to handle tasks such as authentication, redirection, and A/B testing

B) Caching all content at the origin server

C) Storing content in multiple geographic locations

D) Encrypting content at the origin

55. Which of the following is the primary goal of **multi-CDN deployments**?

A) Improving performance by reducing single points of failure and latency

B) Ensuring that content is cached on every edge server

C) Increasing complexity of content delivery

D) Enhancing content security via encryption

56. How does **edge node replication** improve CDN performance?

A) By creating multiple copies of content across different regions to reduce latency

B) By reducing the amount of data that needs to be cached

C) By increasing the number of origin servers

D) By compressing content before it is delivered

57. Which of the following best describes **load balancing at the edge** in CDN systems?

A) Distributing incoming requests among multiple edge servers to optimize resource use and reduce latency

B) Encrypting content during delivery

C) Storing all content in one central location

D) Reducing the number of edge nodes used

58. What is the advantage of using **HTTP/3** in CDNs?

A) Reduced latency by using QUIC protocol, which improves performance on unreliable networks

B) Increased security through better encryption

C) More efficient content compression

D) Enhanced caching capabilities

59. What does **traffic throttling** in a CDN involve?

A) Limiting the amount of traffic that can access certain content to prevent overloads

B) Compressing content for faster delivery

C) Encrypting traffic for security purposes

D) Storing content in multiple edge locations

60. Which CDN feature helps to optimize the delivery of **personalized content**?

A) Dynamic caching and content customization at the edge

B) Using a single content delivery network

C) Pre-fetching all content

D) Encrypting personalized content

61. Why is **real-time traffic monitoring** important in CDN optimization?

A) It helps detect bottlenecks and allows for dynamic adjustments to content delivery

B) It encrypts all incoming and outgoing traffic

C) It reduces the need for edge caching

D) It simplifies the configuration of the origin server

62. Which CDN optimization method is used to enhance **security** in content delivery?

A) Using DDoS protection at the edge

B) Encrypting all content at the origin

C) Increasing cache TTL

D) Storing dynamic content only

63. How do CDN providers optimize **traffic routes**?

A) By selecting the best paths based on real-time network conditions and user location

B) By reducing the number of edge servers used

C) By compressing content for faster delivery

D) By relying on a single origin server

64. Which of the following is a key **optimization goal** for CDN systems in media delivery?

A) Minimizing buffering and improving playback quality

B) Compressing all content to reduce file size

C) Disabling caching to ensure real-time delivery

D) Encrypting content during transmission

65. What role does **load balancing** play in **multi-CDN strategies**?

A) It directs traffic across multiple CDN providers to improve reliability and reduce failure risk

B) It reduces the number of requests to edge servers

C) It caches content across every edge server

D) It encrypts all traffic

66. What is **cache pre-warming** used for in CDNs?

A) Preloading content into caches to ensure fast delivery when users request it

B) Increasing TTL for content

C) Compressing content for quicker delivery

D) Encrypting content before caching

67. How does **HTTP/2** improve CDN performance for dynamic content delivery?

A) By reducing connection setup time and enabling multiplexing of multiple requests

B) By increasing security through encryption

C) By compressing all content before delivery

D) By caching all dynamic content at edge servers

68. Which feature of CDNs helps minimize the effects of **network congestion** during high-traffic events?

A) Real-time traffic management and adaptive routing

B) Enabling content encryption

C) Storing content exclusively at the origin server

D) Using static content for all user requests

69. In a CDN, **edge server health checks** are important because they:

A) Ensure that only healthy edge nodes handle user requests to improve reliability

B) Enable content compression

C) Increase caching TTL for high-priority content

D) Optimize DNS routing for faster access

70. Which strategy in **multi-CDN deployments** helps reduce the **risk of failure**?

A) Intelligent traffic steering and failover to another CDN provider during outages

B) Increasing cache TTL across all CDNs

C) Storing only static content across multiple CDNs

D) Routing all traffic through a single CDN

71. How do CDNs use **edge analytics** to optimize performance?

A) By processing and analyzing user requests at the edge before routing to origin servers

B) By caching all content at the origin server

C) By encrypting all user requests

D) By managing DNS routing in real-time

72. What is the benefit of **decentralized content delivery** in CDNs?

A) It reduces the risk of bottlenecks and improves content delivery speed by distributing traffic to multiple edge locations

B) It centralizes content storage to improve performance

C) It increases encryption of content

D) It simplifies the CDN configuration

73. Which of the following is the main purpose of **edge server isolation** in a CDN?

A) To isolate and secure traffic from malicious requests while delivering content to end users

B) To cache content at the origin server

C) To store user data for later processing

D) To compress content before delivery

74 What does **adaptive content delivery** mean in the context of a CDN?

A) Dynamically adjusting content based on device, network conditions, and user behavior

B) Storing content in multiple edge locations

C) Encrypting all content at the edge

D) Using static content for all users

75. Which technique helps optimize **video content delivery** over a CDN?

A) Adaptive bitrate streaming based on network conditions

B) Compressing video content for faster delivery

C) Increasing the TTL of video content in edge caches

D) Encrypting video files before delivery

76. What is the main advantage of using **Content Delivery Network (CDN) providers** with **global edge presence**?

A) Better performance due to content caching closer to end users, regardless of location

B) Increased content security through global encryption

C) Simplified content management

D) Higher costs due to increased traffic

77. In a CDN, **traffic shaping** techniques are used to:

A) Control the flow of traffic to avoid congestion and optimize delivery

B) Encrypt all incoming traffic

C) Compress data for storage

D) Store content exclusively at edge servers

78. How does **content pre-positioning** work in CDNs to improve performance?

A) It preloads and caches content at strategic locations before user requests, reducing latency

B) It reduces the number of edge servers used

C) It increases the TTL for all cached content

D) It prevents content from being cached

79. Why is **data locality** important in a CDN?

A) It allows content to be cached and delivered more efficiently by keeping it closer to the users' physical locations

B) It increases content encryption

C) It reduces cache evictions

D) It compresses content before delivery

80. What is **serverless computing** in CDN architecture used for?

A) To run code at the edge without requiring traditional server infrastructure, reducing latency

B) To store more content at the origin server

C) To compress content before delivery

D) To improve content encryption

81. How can **cloud-native CDNs** help optimize content delivery for mobile users?

A) By enabling faster content delivery through cloud infrastructure and mobile-specific optimizations

B) By caching all content exclusively at edge servers

C) By storing content at the origin server

D) By encrypting mobile traffic

82. Which of the following is an important benefit of **network optimization** for **video streaming** over CDNs?

A) Improved video quality and reduced buffering by dynamically adjusting to network conditions

B) Increased video file sizes

C) Reduced content encryption

D) Storing all video content in a centralized server

83. What does **cache purging** enable in CDN systems?

A) Removing outdated or invalid content from caches to make room for fresh content

B) Compressing content before caching

C) Storing all content at the origin server

D) Increasing cache TTL for all content

84. How does **multi-layer caching** improve CDN performance for large-scale content delivery?

A) By caching content at different layers (e.g., edge, regional, and origin servers), optimizing access times

B) By compressing all content

C) By limiting the number of edge nodes

D) By encrypting all content before storage

85. What does **real-time optimization** in CDNs refer to?

A) Adjusting content delivery strategies in real-time based on network and user conditions

B) Compressing all content

C) Increasing TTL values for all cached content

D) Encrypting traffic during delivery

86. What is **content fragmentation** in CDNs?

A) Breaking large content files into smaller chunks that can be delivered more efficiently

B) Storing content in multiple locations for redundancy

C) Compressing content to reduce file size

D) Dividing content into smaller pieces for encryption

87. Why is **edge server scaling** important in CDNs?

A) It ensures the network can handle increased traffic and demand by adding more resources to edge nodes

B) It reduces the need for cache purging

C) It improves content compression

D) It increases the amount of content encrypted

88. How do CDNs use **DNS-based load balancing** for traffic management?

A) By directing user requests to the nearest or best-performing edge server based on DNS resolution

B) By compressing content before routing

C) By encrypting all traffic at the DNS level

D) By increasing TTL for DNS records

89. **What does **cache segmentation** enable in CDN configurations?

A) Efficiently handling content based on type, frequency, and geographic location for optimized caching

B) Encrypting content before caching

C) Storing only static content

D) Increasing cache TTL for all content

90. How does **real-time traffic monitoring** support **CDN performance optimization**?

A) By providing insights into traffic trends and enabling adjustments to routing, caching, and load balancing

B) By reducing the number of edge nodes used

C) By compressing all traffic before transmission

D) By improving content security through encryption

91. What is the role of **adaptive bitrate streaming** in video delivery optimization over CDNs?

A) It adjusts the video quality dynamically based on available bandwidth, ensuring smooth playback

B) It increases the file size of videos

C) It caches content at edge servers

D) It encrypts all video content

92. Why is **load balancing** necessary for **multi-CDN environments**?

A) To distribute traffic across multiple CDNs to reduce the risk of failure and improve performance

B) To increase the TTL of cached content

C) To compress all content

D) To store content at the origin server

93. How do **edge cache policies** optimize content delivery?

A) By applying caching rules based on content type, user behavior, and traffic patterns

B) By storing all content at the origin server

C) By compressing content before storage

D) By encrypting content before delivery

94. What role do **analytics** play in CDN optimization?

A) They provide insights into traffic patterns, user behavior, and performance metrics for continuous optimization

B) They compress and encrypt content

C) They increase the TTL for cached content

D) They simplify DNS routing

95. What does **geographic routing** do in a CDN?

A) Routes user requests to the nearest edge server based on geographic location to reduce latency

B) Compresses content based on user location

C) Encrypts content during routing

D) Increases cache TTL for all content

96. What is the key benefit of **real-time load balancing** for CDN performance?

A) Distributing traffic intelligently across edge servers based on current network conditions and traffic volume

B) Encrypting all traffic before routing

C) Caching dynamic content only

D) Compressing content for faster transmission

97. What is **predictive caching** in CDN strategies?

A) Caching content based on predicted user behavior and traffic patterns to reduce cache misses

B) Compressing content before caching

C) Encrypting content before caching

D) Using static content only

98. Which of the following best describes **serverless CDN** architecture?

A) Executing code at the edge without relying on traditional server infrastructure, reducing latency

B) Storing all content at the origin server

C) Compressing content before transmission

D) Encrypting content at the origin

99. What does **content optimization** focus on in CDN architecture?

A) Enhancing delivery speed, reducing latency, and ensuring content is tailored for specific users or devices

B) Storing content in a centralized data center

C) Encrypting all content for security

D) Increasing TTL for all cached content

100. Why is **edge security** important in CDN systems?

A) It protects user data and mitigates DDoS attacks by filtering malicious traffic before it reaches the origin server

B) It compresses all content before delivery

C) It stores content securely at the origin server

D) It encrypts all content at the edge

CDN Use Cases and Industry Applications

1. Which industry benefits most from using a CDN for delivering video content to users?

A) E-commerce

B) Media and entertainment

C) Financial services

D) Healthcare

2. How does a CDN benefit an e-commerce website?

A) By reducing the cost of web hosting

B) By speeding up content delivery and improving user experience

C) By storing large product catalogs on origin servers

D) By compressing all product images

3. Which of the following is a key advantage of using a CDN for global website optimization?

A) Lower website development costs

B) Reduced latency and faster loading times for users worldwide

C) Improved web design capabilities

D) More accurate SEO ranking for local searches

4. What is a common CDN use case in the gaming industry?

A) Reducing the size of game assets

B) Reducing latency for multiplayer gaming experiences

C) Increasing in-app purchases

D) Compressing audio files in games

5. How does a CDN improve the user experience for a media streaming platform?

A) By reducing the cost of streaming licenses

B) By ensuring video content is cached closer to the end user

C) By storing all content in a single data center

D) By enabling faster file downloads for offline viewing

6. Which of the following is a key CDN use case in mobile app delivery?

A) Storing app source code at the origin server

B) Accelerating the delivery of static assets like images, videos, and scripts

C) Encrypting app data in real-time

D) Compressing app data for faster app launches

7. How does a CDN help SaaS (Software as a Service) applications?

A) By reducing the overall cost of cloud infrastructure

B) By ensuring faster response times for users, regardless of location

C) By storing all user data at the origin server

D) By providing unlimited storage options for the application

8. What is the role of a CDN in e-learning platforms?

A) Reducing video resolution for faster playback

B) Caching and delivering educational videos and interactive content faster

C) Compressing all educational resources

D) Preventing access to online learning resources

9. Which of the following industries most commonly uses CDN services for delivering live broadcasts and events?

A) Real estate

B) Media and broadcasting

C) Banking

D) Automotive

10. How do CDNs assist with content delivery for news websites?

A) By distributing breaking news content across multiple edge locations

B) By ensuring all news articles are published to the origin server

C) By reducing website interactivity

D) By increasing the frequency of news article updates

11. Why would a CDN be beneficial for a global e-commerce site during high-traffic events such as Black Friday?

A) By storing user account data at the origin server

B) By balancing the load and ensuring fast, reliable access to product pages worldwide

C) By encrypting payment data in real-time

D) By increasing server capacity to handle requests

12. What role do CDNs play in the delivery of APIs in SaaS applications?

A) By encrypting API responses before sending them to clients

B) By optimizing the routing of API requests to ensure fast and reliable access

C) By restricting access to APIs for security

D) By reducing the number of API requests

13. How do CDNs help with mobile gaming applications?

A) By storing game assets on mobile devices

B) By reducing latency for real-time multiplayer gaming experiences

C) By increasing the file size of the game

D) By compressing game assets before delivery

14. How do CDNs benefit cloud-based applications?

A) By improving access speed to cloud storage

B) By offloading content delivery to edge servers closer to the users

C) By increasing the need for cloud server infrastructure

D) By limiting cloud service access

15. Why would a financial services website use a CDN?

A) To improve the encryption of financial transactions

B) To optimize the delivery of real-time market data and reports globally

C) To reduce the number of transactions processed per day

D) To store all financial data at a single central location

16. Which industry benefits from using CDNs for software updates and patches?

A) Gaming

B) Healthcare

C) Retail

D) Cybersecurity

17. In which scenario would a CDN be used to optimize content delivery for a healthcare portal?

A) Speeding up the delivery of medical resources, patient information, and educational content

B) Compressing medical records for storage

C) Encrypting medical data in real-time

D) Reducing the load on origin servers

18. How does a CDN enhance the performance of a streaming video platform during high traffic periods?

A) By compressing video files in real-time

B) By distributing content across edge servers to reduce latency and buffering

C) By encrypting all user data

D) By storing videos only on a single server

19. What is the benefit of using a CDN for the delivery of multimedia content on news websites?

A) Improved SEO rankings

B) Faster delivery of images, videos, and other rich media to users worldwide

C) Reducing the need for interactive content

D) Minimizing the cost of content creation

20. Which of the following industries uses CDNs to ensure fast and secure delivery of high-value transactions?

A) E-commerce

B) Banking and finance

C) Social media

D) Education

21. How do CDNs help ensure that websites can handle traffic spikes from social media campaigns?

A) By compressing all images and videos in real-time

B) By delivering content from multiple distributed edge locations

C) By limiting the number of requests processed

D) By using cloud-based storage only

22. In which case would a CDN optimize content delivery for IoT (Internet of Things) applications?

A) By increasing the number of devices connected to the network

B) By improving latency for real-time device-to-device communication

C) By reducing the need for edge server infrastructure

D) By compressing IoT data during transmission

23. How does a CDN help with the global delivery of advertisements?

A) By caching and delivering ad content based on geographic location and user behavior

B) By compressing all ads for faster delivery

C) By storing ads only at the origin server

D) By encrypting ad content for security

24. Why do e-commerce sites use CDNs to deliver product images and videos?

A) To store them in a centralized server location

B) To ensure faster and more reliable loading times for users worldwide

C) To reduce the file size of images

D) To provide better SEO rankings

25. Which of the following is a major benefit of using a CDN for a live event streaming website?

A) Reducing video resolution to save bandwidth

B) Delivering high-quality video content with minimal buffering for viewers worldwide

C) Compressing live streams for faster transmission

D) Storing live events at the origin server for security

26. How does a CDN assist with optimizing delivery for online gaming?

A) By reducing the size of game files

B) By ensuring fast content delivery to reduce latency in multiplayer gaming sessions

C) By compressing game assets

D) By caching all game assets at the origin server

27. What role do CDNs play in the performance of video-on-demand services?

A) Reducing the resolution of videos to save bandwidth

B) Caching videos at edge servers to ensure faster start times and reduce buffering

C) Encrypting all videos for security

D) Storing all videos at a centralized server

28. How does a CDN support faster content delivery for a global e-learning platform?

A) By compressing all videos for faster playback

B) By caching video lessons and resources close to learners' geographic locations

C) By restricting access to educational content

D) By reducing the resolution of educational videos

29. Which industry benefits from using a CDN to accelerate the delivery of critical weather data to users?

A) Finance

B) Travel and transportation

C) Telecommunications

D) Healthcare

30. What is the main benefit of using CDNs for real-time sports streaming platforms?

A) Reduced video quality

B) Faster content delivery to reduce latency and buffering during live events

C) Compressing live streams for storage

D) Limiting access to live broadcasts

31. Why is a CDN crucial for social media platforms?

A) To compress all user-uploaded images and videos

B) To deliver user-generated content like images, videos, and posts to users with minimal latency

C) To reduce the file size of videos and images

D) To limit video resolution

32. Which CDN strategy is most commonly used by media companies for distributing their content globally?

A) Multi-CDN setup to improve reliability

B) Limiting content delivery to only one region

C) Centralizing all content storage

D) Compressing all video files to reduce bandwidth

33. How do CDNs support financial trading platforms?

A) By reducing the latency of stock price updates and improving the speed of transaction processing

B) By compressing financial reports for faster delivery

C) By securing all data transmissions

D) By limiting access to financial data

34. In which scenario would a CDN help improve the user experience for a live news feed website?

A) By storing all content on a central server

B) By delivering content faster by caching news articles at edge servers

C) By reducing the quality of news content

D) By compressing content for transmission

35. How does a CDN assist with the delivery of digital media content for a music streaming service?

A) By encrypting all music tracks for security

B) By caching music tracks and delivering them from the nearest edge server to reduce latency

C) By compressing all audio files

D) By storing music files only on a centralized server

36. Why do content publishers use CDNs to serve their digital advertisements?

A) To increase the load time of ads

B) To ensure faster and more efficient delivery of ads to users globally

C) To prevent ads from being blocked by browsers

D) To store ads only at the origin server

37. How does a CDN help improve the performance of an international e-commerce platform during flash sales?

A) By storing all product images in the cloud

B) By optimizing content delivery, ensuring low latency and fast loading times during high-traffic events

C) By reducing the cost of infrastructure

D) By compressing product images and videos for storage

38. In a CDN, how do edge servers help optimize content delivery for users in remote or underserved regions?

A) By storing content only at the origin server

B) By caching and delivering content from servers closer to the user, reducing latency

C) By increasing the size of the content

D) By compressing content before storing it

39. Which of the following is a key benefit of using CDNs for real-time data feeds (e.g., financial or IoT data)?

A) Increased encryption of data feeds

B) Faster data transmission by caching data close to users and reducing network hops

C) Storing all data in a centralized location

D) Compressing data feeds for smaller file sizes

40. Why are CDNs important for global travel and tourism websites?

A) To compress all travel photos

B) To cache destination information, booking systems, and images closer to global users, ensuring fast access

C) To limit access to only specific regions

D) To store all content in one centralized location

41. How does a CDN benefit online advertising platforms?

A) By encrypting all ads for security

B) By delivering ad content more quickly, reducing latency, and improving ad viewability

C) By restricting the number of ad impressions per user

D) By reducing the overall ad budget

42. What role do CDNs play in optimizing the delivery of media content on social media platforms?

A) By caching videos and images at edge servers, ensuring faster load times for users globally

B) By limiting the number of social media posts displayed to users

C) By reducing the quality of images and videos

D) By encrypting user data

43. In which scenario would a CDN benefit the delivery of software downloads for a global user base?

A) By reducing the size of the software installation package

B) By storing the software packages closer to users for faster and more reliable downloads

C) By limiting the number of users allowed to download the software

D) By compressing all software packages for smaller file sizes

44. How does a CDN improve the performance of video conferencing platforms?

A) By compressing video data for faster delivery

B) By reducing the video resolution

C) By caching video streams at edge locations to reduce latency and ensure smoother video calls

D) By limiting the number of video participants per call

45. Which of the following is a key reason why cloud gaming platforms use CDNs?

A) To increase the file size of game assets

B) To reduce latency and improve the responsiveness of game data for users around the world

C) To store all game assets in a centralized location

D) To compress all game assets for faster transmission

46. How do CDNs help optimize the delivery of interactive content on e-learning platforms?

A) By compressing all interactive elements

B) By caching and delivering interactive media, quizzes, and videos closer to the learner's geographic location

C) By reducing the resolution of videos

D) By limiting access to certain course content

47. What is the advantage of using CDNs for cloud-based video streaming services during peak usage times?

A) By storing videos at the origin server for quick access

B) By caching and distributing video content across multiple edge servers to ensure a smooth and uninterrupted experience

C) By compressing videos before delivery

D) By encrypting all video files

48. Why would a CDN be used for a digital marketing agency managing client campaigns globally?

A) To store client data in one centralized server

B) To ensure fast, reliable delivery of marketing content (e.g., ads, landing pages, media) to users worldwide

C) To reduce the number of marketing campaigns created

D) To compress marketing content for faster transmission

49. How does a CDN improve the performance of a news website during breaking news events?

A) By storing all news content at a centralized server

B) By delivering breaking news content quickly to users through caching at edge servers

C) By reducing the quality of content during high-traffic events

D) By encrypting all news articles for security

50. How do CDNs help online education platforms scale during massive course enrollments?

A) By limiting the number of course access points

B) By caching educational content (videos, materials) closer to students' locations, reducing load on central servers

C) By compressing educational content for faster delivery

D) By restricting access to course materials during peak periods

51. What is the benefit of using CDNs for the delivery of mobile apps in the App Store or Google Play?

A) By reducing the number of app updates available

B) By ensuring faster and more efficient downloads by caching app packages at edge servers

C) By compressing app code

D) By limiting the number of downloads per user

52. Which industry benefits the most from CDNs for accelerating content delivery during live auctions and bidding events?

A) Healthcare

B) E-commerce

C) Art and collectibles

D) Finance

53. How do CDNs help ensure the high availability of content during peak shopping seasons (e.g., Cyber Monday)?

A) By compressing all product images and videos

B) By balancing the load and distributing traffic across multiple edge servers to reduce bottlenecks

C) By storing all product inventory at the origin server

D) By limiting access to product pages

54. What is the key advantage of using CDNs in the healthcare industry for delivering medical content?

A) Reducing file sizes for medical reports

B) Ensuring faster and more secure delivery of medical resources and educational content to professionals and patients globally

C) Encrypting patient data at the edge

D) Storing medical data only on the origin server

55. How does a CDN optimize content delivery for an e-commerce site with multiple product categories?

A) By delivering product images, videos, and catalogs from multiple edge servers, ensuring fast loading times across regions

B) By limiting product selection based on region

C) By compressing product content to reduce file sizes

D) By storing all product information in a single location

56. How does a CDN support the rapid delivery of product reviews on e-commerce websites?

A) By limiting access to product reviews

B) By caching and delivering reviews close to the user, improving load times and user interaction

C) By compressing review text

D) By storing all reviews at the origin server

57. How does a CDN help with the delivery of mobile content on a website optimized for smartphones?

A) By compressing all mobile content for faster delivery

B) By serving optimized versions of images and videos tailored to mobile users from the nearest edge server

C) By reducing the size of mobile websites

D) By increasing the number of mobile app downloads

58. How does a CDN enhance security for a global e-commerce website?

A) By encrypting user data during delivery

B) By reducing the risk of DDoS attacks and protecting user data through edge security features

C) By limiting the number of international users accessing the site

D) By compressing content before delivery

59. What role does a CDN play in delivering real-time updates on sports websites?

A) It reduces the resolution of live sports videos

B) It caches live score updates and video streams at edge locations for faster delivery to users globally

C) It compresses all sports video content

D) It restricts live sports broadcasts to specific geographic regions

60. How do CDNs benefit the delivery of highly dynamic content, such as personalized web pages or user dashboards?

A) By caching all dynamic content and reducing the need for frequent server requests

B) By caching static content only

C) By storing all user data in a central location

D) By encrypting user dashboards in real-time

61. What is the role of a CDN in the performance of online ticket booking platforms?

A) By delivering high-demand content (e.g., event details, ticket availability) faster through caching at edge servers

B) By storing all ticketing data at the origin server

C) By compressing event images for faster delivery

D) By limiting access to tickets during peak times

62. How do CDNs improve performance for video-on-demand platforms during simultaneous global usage?

A) By reducing video quality

B) By caching video files at edge servers around the world to ensure fast, smooth playback for users

C) By increasing server capacity

D) By restricting access to high-demand content

63. How do CDNs benefit websites that rely on real-time user-generated content, such as social media platforms?

A) By restricting user access based on region

B) By caching and delivering user-generated content (images, videos, posts) quickly to global users

C) By compressing all user-uploaded media

D) By storing all user content on a central server

64. Which industry benefits from CDNs for securely delivering confidential data in real-time, such as legal documents or contracts?

A) Retail

B) Legal services

C) Healthcare

D) Finance

65. Why do travel agencies use CDNs to optimize the delivery of travel information on their websites?

A) To ensure faster access to booking systems and destination content by users worldwide

B) To reduce the number of available travel destinations

C) To compress travel images for storage

D) To store all travel information at a centralized data center

66. How does a CDN assist in reducing the impact of network congestion for media streaming services?

A) By increasing the size of content

B) By storing video content closer to users on edge servers, bypassing congested backbone networks

C) By compressing video content in real-time

D) By limiting access to high-definition content

67. In the context of CDN use for e-commerce, how can CDNs improve the performance of search functionality on large retail websites?

A) By reducing the number of products displayed

B) By caching frequently searched queries and product information to speed up search results

C) By compressing search results

D) By storing all search data at the origin server

68. How does a CDN enhance the user experience for a SaaS (Software as a Service) platform that serves dynamic, personalized content?

A) By storing all user data at the origin server

B) By caching personalized content based on user preferences and delivering it from the nearest edge server

C) By compressing personalized content before delivery

D) By restricting the number of users accessing the platform

69. How do CDNs help with global performance optimization for a website that targets customers in both Asia and North America?

A) By storing all content in a single location in North America

B) By caching content at edge locations in both regions, ensuring faster load times regardless of the user's location

C) By limiting access to certain regions

D) By compressing content for smaller file sizes

70. Why are CDNs particularly beneficial for global media content distribution, such as movie streaming services?

A) By reducing the resolution of videos to save bandwidth

B) By caching and delivering high-quality video content from servers closer to viewers, reducing buffering and latency

C) By encrypting video streams in real-time

D) By storing all video content at the origin server

71. In what way does a CDN help reduce the strain on the origin server for high-traffic websites like online ticket booking platforms?

A) By storing all transaction data at the edge

B) By caching and serving static content, reducing the load on the origin server and preventing bottlenecks

C) By compressing transaction data

D) By limiting access to tickets during peak periods

72. How do CDNs improve content delivery for a digital publishing company that serves millions of readers worldwide?

A) By storing all articles at the origin server

B) By caching articles and media at edge locations and ensuring fast, reliable access for readers worldwide

C) By compressing articles for faster delivery

D) By limiting access to certain content

73. Which of the following industries benefits from CDNs in delivering digital advertising content in real-time?

A) Healthcare

B) Marketing and advertising

C) Retail

D) Education

74. Why would a video game streaming platform use a CDN for game streaming?

A) To store games at a centralized server

B) To reduce latency and buffering by delivering game streams from edge locations closer to the user

C) To compress game streams in real-time

D) To limit the number of game streams available

75. How do CDNs support the global distribution of large software files, such as operating system updates?

A) By limiting download sizes

B) By caching software updates at edge servers to improve download speeds and reduce strain on origin servers

C) By compressing software updates to reduce download size

D) By storing all software updates at the origin server

76. How do CDNs enhance the performance of live streaming platforms during high-traffic events, such as concerts or sports games?

A) By reducing video resolution

B) By distributing live streams across multiple edge locations, ensuring smoother playback and less buffering for viewers worldwide

C) By compressing video content in real-time

D) By storing live streams only at the origin server

77. What is one of the main reasons e-commerce businesses use CDNs to accelerate page load times for product pages?

A) To store images in a centralized data center

B) To reduce the number of product images and descriptions displayed

C) To cache product images, descriptions, and other static content, improving page load times for customers worldwide

D) To compress product images for faster delivery

78. Why do CDN providers offer security features like DDoS protection for high-traffic websites?

A) To reduce the number of website visitors

B) To ensure websites remain operational during cyber-attacks by filtering malicious traffic before it reaches the origin server

C) To compress all website content

D) To restrict access to certain website pages

79. How does a CDN benefit the performance of an interactive online gaming platform?

A) By reducing the number of active users

B) By caching game assets at edge servers and delivering them faster, improving the gaming experience for users worldwide

C) By compressing game files

D) By limiting real-time gameplay features

80. How do CDNs assist in optimizing content delivery for online news aggregators during breaking news events?

A) By reducing the number of news stories published

B) By caching and delivering news content from edge servers close to readers to ensure quick updates during high-traffic periods

C) By encrypting all news articles

D) By limiting access to specific news stories

81. Why would a CDN be beneficial for a healthcare portal that delivers medical videos and educational content?

A) By compressing medical videos

B) By caching and delivering educational videos, articles, and other content closer to medical professionals and patients globally

C) By limiting the types of medical content available

D) By storing all medical content in a centralized location

82. How do CDNs enhance the user experience for a global travel booking platform?

A) By restricting access to booking pages

B) By caching travel information, images, and booking forms at edge servers, ensuring fast access regardless of the user's location

C) By reducing the number of destinations available to users

D) By compressing travel images for storage

83. How does a CDN help video-on-demand platforms handle large traffic spikes during new content releases?

A) By reducing the video resolution for users

B) By caching new video content at edge locations to ensure smooth, high-quality streaming during high-traffic periods

C) By limiting video availability during peak hours

D) By compressing all video content

84. How do CDNs assist global advertising networks in delivering ads to users based on geographic location?

A) By compressing ads for faster delivery

B) By caching ads at edge servers and ensuring they are tailored to user interests and geographic locations

C) By reducing the number of ads delivered

D) By storing ads only at the origin server

85. Why would a CDN be beneficial for a SaaS company that provides a customer portal?

A) By storing all customer data at a centralized server

B) By caching and delivering dynamic content like personalized dashboards faster, reducing latency for global users

C) By compressing dynamic content for delivery

D) By restricting user access to certain portal features

86. How do CDNs help accelerate content delivery for real-time collaborative platforms, like online document editing?

A) By compressing real-time content updates

B) By caching document versions at edge servers, ensuring quick access and synchronization between collaborators

C) By limiting the number of collaborators per document

D) By reducing the number of document changes allowed

87. How do CDNs optimize the performance of a global stock trading platform?

A) By compressing stock price data

B) By caching real-time stock prices and financial news to ensure low-latency delivery to traders worldwide

C) By limiting the number of stock transactions per minute

D) By storing financial data at the origin server

88. How does a CDN improve the delivery of user reviews and ratings for products on an e-commerce site?

A) By storing all reviews in a centralized database

B) By caching product reviews and ratings closer to users, ensuring fast load times for product pages

C) By compressing user reviews

D) By limiting the number of reviews displayed on each page

89. How do CDNs enhance content delivery for interactive and multimedia-rich websites, such as online education or virtual tours?

A) By reducing the quality of multimedia content

B) By caching interactive media (images, videos, virtual tours) close to the user for faster delivery and smoother interaction

C) By storing content only on a central server

D) By limiting the multimedia content available during high traffic times

90. How does a CDN support the delivery of high-volume news video content on a global scale?

A) By reducing video resolution

B) By caching video content at multiple edge locations, ensuring smooth and efficient delivery of news broadcasts worldwide

C) By compressing news video for storage

D) By restricting access to video content based on region

91. How does a CDN benefit a global e-learning platform with a large student base in various countries?

A) By storing all course content in one centralized location

B) By caching and delivering course videos, quizzes, and other materials from the nearest edge server to reduce latency and improve accessibility

C) By limiting access to courses based on geographic regions

D) By compressing course content for storage

92. Why is a CDN essential for delivering real-time notifications for a global sports app?

A) By encrypting notifications for added security

B) By caching notifications at edge servers to ensure timely delivery of real-time scores, updates, and alerts to users worldwide

C) By limiting the number of notifications sent per user

D) By compressing notification content

93. In which scenario would a CDN optimize the performance of an online auction platform?

A) By storing auction data at the origin server

B) By caching auction details (e.g., bids, items, countdown timers) and serving them from the nearest edge servers to reduce latency during live auctions

C) By compressing auction images

D) By limiting the number of users participating in an auction

94. How do CDNs help with the delivery of high-volume transactional data, such as order confirmations and invoices, for global e-commerce websites?

A) By encrypting all transactional data

B) By caching order confirmations and invoices at edge locations, ensuring that these pages load quickly for global customers

C) By compressing transactional data for faster transmission

D) By storing transactional data only at the origin server

95. Why are CDNs useful for improving the delivery of customer support content, such as knowledge bases and FAQs, on global websites?

A) By storing all support content in a single location

B) By caching and delivering support articles, FAQs, and guides from the nearest edge servers, ensuring faster access for users worldwide

C) By reducing the quality of the content

D) By limiting access to certain support pages

96. What is the main reason a CDN is used to serve high-definition video content for a global audience?

A) To compress video content for faster delivery

B) To cache and deliver video content from servers closer to the user's location, ensuring smooth playback and minimal buffering

C) To limit access to specific video formats

D) To reduce the video resolution during peak times

97. How does a CDN help e-commerce websites improve the checkout process during peak traffic times?

A) By compressing all transaction data

B) By caching product pages, images, and checkout pages at edge servers, reducing the load on origin servers and speeding up the checkout process

C) By limiting access to checkout features

D) By storing all transaction data at the origin server

98. Why do financial services platforms use CDNs for delivering real-time stock quotes and trading data?

A) By caching financial data at edge servers, enabling low-latency access to stock quotes and trading information globally

B) By encrypting all stock quote data

C) By compressing financial reports for storage

D) By storing stock data only at the origin server

99. How does a CDN support the delivery of global marketing campaigns, such as ad banners or promotional content?

A) By reducing the size of ad banners

B) By caching ad content closer to the user's location and ensuring faster loading times for global audiences

C) By limiting the number of marketing campaigns served

D) By storing all ad content on a single server

100. How do CDNs benefit online video-sharing platforms like YouTube or Vimeo during periods of viral content popularity?

A) By limiting access to viral videos

B) By caching and distributing viral video content to edge locations, ensuring that it can be accessed quickly and smoothly by viewers worldwide without overloading central servers

C) By compressing video files for smaller sizes

D) By storing all videos at the origin server

Case Studies of CDN Success

1. **What was one of the primary reasons for Netflix's successful global expansion using a CDN?**

   A) They only used servers in North America

   B) They reduced video resolution globally

   C) They cached content closer to users, reducing buffering and improving streaming quality

   D) They compressed video content for smaller file sizes

2. **How did Spotify leverage CDNs to improve the user experience?**

   A) By streaming all music from a single origin server

   B) By caching music tracks and playlists at edge servers, reducing load times for users worldwide

   C) By offering limited song choices to users in certain regions

   D) By reducing the quality of the music streams during peak usage

3. **Which of the following best describes how CDNs helped Amazon during Black Friday sales?**

   A) By limiting access to some product categories

   B) By offloading static content (like images and descriptions) to edge servers to handle massive traffic spikes

   C) By restricting access to certain regions during peak times

   D) By reducing the number of product options available during the sale

4. **Why did the BBC use a CDN for the delivery of their iPlayer streaming service?**

   A) To restrict access to content based on user location

   B) To cache live and on-demand video content close to users, reducing buffering and improving playback quality

   C) To compress all video content

   D) To store all video content at a central data center

5. **How did a global CDN help global e-commerce giant eBay scale their platform during high-traffic events like Cyber Monday?**

   A) By restricting access to certain products

B) By offloading static content (like images and descriptions) to edge servers, reducing latency during peak traffic times

C) By compressing all content on the site

D) By limiting the number of items available for purchase

6. **What role did CDNs play in supporting YouTube's global success?**

A) By storing videos on a central server

B) By caching videos on multiple edge servers around the world, ensuring smooth playback even during high-traffic events

C) By limiting video resolution globally

D) By streaming content from a single data center in North America

7. **How did Akamai CDN benefit Adobe's cloud services platform?**

A) By compressing all files uploaded by users

B) By reducing the number of users accessing Adobe's platform

C) By speeding up the delivery of software updates, content, and creative assets for Adobe Creative Cloud users worldwide

D) By limiting access to certain features

8. **Why did Stack Overflow use a CDN to accelerate content delivery for its global developer community?**

A) By limiting access to questions based on location

B) By caching frequently accessed content, such as questions and answers, to improve site load times across different regions

C) By compressing all content uploaded by users

D) By storing all data at a central server

9. **How did Shopify benefit from implementing a CDN in its e-commerce platform?**

A) By restricting the number of products on the website

B) By caching product images, descriptions, and other assets to reduce latency for global shoppers

C) By reducing the number of active users accessing the platform

D) By limiting product variations for faster load times

10. **Which company used CDNs to ensure a smooth video streaming experience during live events like the Olympics?**

A) Facebook

B) Netflix

C) NBC Universal

D) Hulu

11. **How did the New York Times use a CDN to improve page load times for its readers around the world?**

A) By limiting access to articles

B) By caching static content like images, headlines, and text to speed up loading times for readers in different regions

C) By reducing the size of article content

D) By compressing images globally

12. **What benefit did a CDN provide for the mobile app of a large airline company?**

A) Reduced the number of available flights per day

B) Cached flight data and customer service content to ensure faster load times and improve customer experience for travelers worldwide

C) Limited the number of users accessing flight information

D) Compressing flight schedules

13. **How did the content delivery network improve the user experience for Disney+?**

A) By reducing video resolution

B) By caching video content at edge servers around the world, ensuring smooth playback of movies and TV shows regardless of location

C) By compressing video files to lower quality

D) By storing all content at a single origin server

14. **Why did the sports streaming platform, FuboTV, choose to use a CDN?**

A) To limit access to certain events

B) To provide faster and more reliable live-streaming of sporting events by caching video content close to the user's location

C) To compress all video streams

D) To reduce the number of viewers per event

15. **Which of the following best describes how CDNs helped CNN during major breaking news events?**

A) By limiting access to certain news stories

B) By caching news stories, videos, and images at edge servers, ensuring fast and reliable delivery during high-traffic events

C) By compressing live news content

D) By restricting live streaming of breaking news

16. **How did CDNs assist in the success of online learning platforms like Coursera?**

A) By reducing the number of courses available to students

B) By caching video lectures, quizzes, and assignments at edge locations to ensure fast and uninterrupted access for students worldwide

C) By compressing course videos

D) By storing all content at a centralized server

17. **How did CDNs help BBC News manage traffic spikes during high-profile events such as elections or royal weddings?**

A) By reducing the number of articles available

B) By caching and distributing news stories and live updates from edge servers, ensuring smooth delivery during traffic spikes

C) By restricting access to some articles

D) By compressing video streams during live broadcasts

18. **How did the CDN optimize performance for the video streaming service, Vimeo?**

A) By streaming content from a single server

B) By caching and delivering video content from edge locations to ensure smoother playback across global regions

C) By reducing the resolution of videos

D) By compressing all video files during delivery

19. **Why did Walmart use a CDN to handle traffic surges during events like Black Friday?**

A) By limiting access to certain products during peak times

B) By caching and distributing product pages, images, and checkout processes from edge servers, ensuring faster load times during high traffic

C) By compressing all product images

D) By restricting access to certain regions

20. **How did the CDN benefit the global music service, Deezer, during traffic spikes?**

A) By storing music files on a central server

B) By caching popular tracks and playlists at edge servers worldwide, ensuring smooth playback during high-traffic times

C) By compressing music files for faster streaming

D) By reducing the number of available songs

21. **How did YouTube improve its service with the use of a CDN for live streaming events?**

A) By storing all live streams at a central data center

B) By caching live video content at edge locations, reducing latency and improving stream stability for global viewers

C) By compressing live video streams

D) By restricting the number of live streams

22. **Which large-scale CDN deployment helped the media company, Turner Broadcasting, handle a massive surge of viewers during the March Madness basketball tournament?**

A) Amazon Web Services (AWS)

B) Akamai

C) Fastly

D) Cloudflare

23. **How did a CDN enable Twitch to improve its streaming platform for gamers worldwide?**

A) By restricting access to gaming streams

B) By caching video game streams at edge servers to ensure smooth and low-latency playback for gamers around the world

C) By reducing video quality globally

D) By limiting the number of active streamers

24. **How did the European Space Agency (ESA) benefit from a CDN during the launch of its spacecraft?**

A) By reducing the number of viewers allowed to watch the event

B) By delivering live-streaming videos of the launch from servers close to viewers, ensuring smooth playback even during high traffic

C) By storing all launch content in one location

D) By compressing video content in real-time

25. **Why did major online education platforms like Khan Academy choose CDNs to optimize content delivery?**

A) To compress educational videos

B) By caching video lessons and interactive content at edge servers, ensuring fast access and reducing buffering for global students

C) By limiting access to lessons during peak times

D) By storing all content in a central location

26. **How did CDN technology help Bloomberg deliver financial data to global markets?**

A) By compressing financial reports

B) By caching stock market updates and financial news at edge servers, ensuring real-time delivery with low latency

C) By limiting access to market data during high volatility

D) By streaming data from a single server location

27. **How did CDNs help Twitch improve live streaming during major eSports events?**

A) By restricting access to certain streams

B) By caching live gaming streams at edge locations to minimize latency and provide high-quality broadcasts to global audiences

C) By reducing video quality during peak traffic times

D) By storing all live streams in a single central location

28. **How did Netflix use a CDN to reduce latency for viewers in regions with slower internet speeds?**

A) By limiting video quality for slower networks

B) By caching video content closer to the user's location, improving streaming speed and reducing buffering for viewers globally

C) By reducing the number of users allowed to watch content in certain regions

D) By compressing all video content

29. **How did Akamai's CDN help Microsoft deliver software updates for Windows?**

A) By limiting the number of users downloading updates

B) By caching update files at edge servers, reducing download times and server load

C) By compressing all software update files

D) By restricting updates to specific geographic regions

30. **Why did Adobe use a CDN for its Creative Cloud services?**

A) To limit the number of users accessing the platform

B) By caching and delivering software updates and creative assets quickly, regardless of the user's location

C) By compressing Creative Cloud assets

D) By restricting access to some creative tools during peak traffic

31. **How did CDNs improve user experience for mobile gaming platforms like PUBG Mobile?**

A) By limiting access to certain regions

B) By caching gaming assets, such as images and maps, at edge servers to reduce load times and latency for players around the world

C) By compressing all gaming data

D) By storing all data in one centralized server

32. **What role did CDNs play in enabling global-scale online multiplayer gaming experiences?**

A) By reducing the number of players in each game session

B) By caching game data and player interactions at edge locations, reducing latency and ensuring smooth gameplay for global players

C) By compressing in-game assets for faster downloads

D) By limiting access to certain game modes

33. **How did CDNs assist with the global distribution of app updates for companies like Apple and Google?**

A) By restricting the number of downloads per day

B) By caching app files at edge servers, speeding up download times and reducing strain on origin servers

C) By compressing app updates for smaller file sizes

D) By limiting access to updates based on device type

34. **How did CDNs benefit the delivery of eBooks and digital publications to users on platforms like Amazon Kindle?**

A) By compressing eBook files

B) By caching digital content and delivering it quickly from edge servers to readers around the world, ensuring fast download speeds

C) By limiting access to certain publications

D) By storing all digital content on a single server

35. **How did a CDN improve the experience of users accessing news websites during breaking events?**

A) By limiting access to some news stories

B) By caching static content (headlines, images) at edge locations, ensuring quick page load times and reducing strain on origin servers during high traffic periods

C) By reducing image resolution during peak times

D) By restricting access to live streams

36. **Why did CNN deploy a CDN to handle global traffic during major events like presidential elections?**

A) To compress live video streams

B) By caching news content, live streams, and updates at multiple edge servers, ensuring reliable delivery despite high traffic volumes

C) By limiting the number of users accessing live content

D) By restricting access to content in certain regions

37. **How did CDNs help with the delivery of content for the online news site, The Guardian?**

A) By restricting access to certain articles

B) By caching images, articles, and videos at edge servers, ensuring faster loading times for readers worldwide

C) By compressing article content

D) By reducing the number of articles available to global users

38. **What was one of the key benefits for an airline using a CDN for its website and app?**

A) Reduced access to booking pages

B) By caching flight and booking information at edge servers, improving website speed and ensuring a smooth experience for travelers worldwide

C) By compressing all booking data

D) By restricting the number of flight routes available

39. **How did CDNs enhance the delivery of digital media for an online education platform like Udemy?**

A) By compressing video courses

B) By caching course videos, tutorials, and learning materials at edge servers, ensuring fast delivery and minimal buffering for students worldwide

C) By limiting the number of courses available

D) By restricting access to certain regions

40. **Why did the video platform Dailymotion implement a CDN for its global video streaming?**

A) By limiting access to specific video formats

B) By caching video content at edge servers globally to improve stream quality and minimize buffering during high traffic events

C) By reducing the video resolution

D) By storing all videos in a single central location

41. **What role did a CDN play in Facebook's delivery of real-time updates and content?**

A) By compressing user posts

B) By caching posts, images, and videos at edge servers, ensuring fast delivery of content to users across the globe

C) By restricting content availability during peak traffic times

D) By storing content only in the United States

42. **How did Spotify optimize music streaming using a CDN?**

A) By compressing music files

B) By caching music files at edge servers to improve streaming speed and reduce buffering for users worldwide

C) By limiting access to certain albums

D) By reducing the quality of streams based on user location

43. **Why did Apple choose to use a CDN for the global delivery of its software updates for macOS and iOS?**

A) To restrict access to updates based on region

B) By caching software updates at edge locations, reducing download times and server load during updates

C) By compressing update files

D) By limiting access to only certain device models

44. **How did a CDN assist in the distribution of video content during the release of a major film via streaming platforms like Amazon Prime Video?**

A) By compressing the video files

B) By caching video content on edge servers around the world, ensuring that users could access the film without interruption regardless of location

C) By reducing the video resolution

D) By limiting the number of users allowed to watch

45. **How did CDNs enable rapid scaling for the global launch of a mobile app on Google Play and the Apple App Store?**

A) By reducing the number of downloads

B) By caching app installation files at multiple edge servers to speed up downloads during high-demand periods

C) By compressing app data

D) By limiting app functionality during high traffic

46. **How did the New York Times use a CDN to ensure timely access to breaking news during high-traffic events like elections?**

A) By compressing all articles and videos

B) By caching articles, videos, and images at edge servers to provide quick access during traffic surges

C) By limiting access to certain news content

D) By reducing the number of visitors allowed to access the site

47. **How did CDNs support the global scalability of the cloud-based video conferencing platform Zoom?**

A) By limiting access to the platform during high-traffic times

B) By caching meeting data, video, and audio files at edge locations, improving call quality and reducing latency for users globally

C) By reducing video resolution during peak usage

D) By compressing audio and video files during meetings

48. **Why did CDNs play an essential role in the success of the live-streaming platform Periscope?**

A) By limiting access to certain streams

B) By caching live video streams at edge servers globally, ensuring smooth real-time broadcasts with minimal latency

C) By compressing all live video content

D) By storing live streams only on central servers

49. **How did CDNs help improve content delivery for the gaming platform Steam?**

A) By compressing game files

B) By caching game downloads and updates at edge servers to reduce latency and ensure faster download speeds for users worldwide

C) By limiting access to certain game updates

D) By reducing the size of game files

50. **How did CDNs enhance the delivery of video content for the National Geographic website?**

A) By compressing videos for faster streaming

B) By caching videos and images at edge servers, improving access speed and reducing buffering for global users

C) By limiting the number of videos available

D) By reducing the quality of videos during peak traffic

51. **How did a CDN benefit the gaming company Riot Games during global launch events?**

A) By limiting the number of active users during the launch

B) By caching gaming assets and in-game content at edge servers, ensuring low-latency gameplay and fast updates for players worldwide

C) By reducing game download sizes

D) By compressing in-game graphics and animations

52. **How did a CDN help the European Union's digital platform, EU Open Data Portal, handle large traffic spikes?**

A) By limiting the number of users accessing the portal

B) By caching static datasets and ensuring faster access to public data across multiple regions in the EU

C) By compressing all data downloads

D) By restricting access to certain datasets based on user region

53. **Why did CDNs help the media company, Hulu, deliver its streaming service effectively?**

A) By limiting the number of streams per user

B) By caching streaming content at edge servers, reducing buffering and ensuring smooth playback for viewers globally

C) By reducing the video resolution

D) By storing content only in the United States

54. **What impact did CDNs have on content delivery for the online video platform, Vimeo, during high-traffic events?**

A) By restricting access to certain video categories

B) By caching videos at edge locations and ensuring seamless streaming for global viewers during large events like film premieres or live concerts

C) By compressing videos during live events

D) By reducing the number of video streams available for users

55. **How did a CDN benefit the delivery of video tutorials on online learning platforms like Lynda.com?**

A) By restricting access to certain tutorials

B) By caching video lessons and other content, ensuring fast and reliable delivery of educational materials to students worldwide

C) By compressing tutorial videos

D) By limiting the number of lessons available during peak usage

56. **Why did the social media network Twitter use a CDN?**

A) To store all content in a single location

B) By caching user-generated content (tweets, images, and videos) at edge locations, ensuring rapid delivery and reducing latency for global users

C) By compressing all tweets and images

D) By restricting access to certain tweets

57. **How did CNN improve user experience for viewers watching live news coverage using a CDN?**

A) By limiting access to live streams

B) By caching live video content and news updates at edge servers, improving the speed and reliability of news delivery to global audiences

C) By compressing all live news streams

D) By reducing the number of articles available for viewing

58. **How did the CDN help facilitate smoother delivery of content for the global e-learning platform, Skillshare?**

A) By reducing the size of video lessons

B) By caching educational videos, assignments, and learning materials at edge servers, providing faster access to students worldwide

C) By limiting the number of students who can access a course at once

D) By compressing interactive content during lessons

59. **How did the CDN help with global delivery for the live streaming service Periscope?**

A) By limiting the number of live streams per event

B) By caching live streaming video feeds at edge locations, ensuring smooth video quality and low latency during high-traffic events

C) By reducing the resolution of live video

D) By compressing live video feeds in real-time

60. **What key benefit did the BBC iPlayer streaming service gain from using a CDN?**

A) By compressing video files

B) By caching live and on-demand videos at edge locations to ensure smooth playback and reduce buffering for viewers worldwide

C) By restricting the resolution of videos based on bandwidth

D) By limiting the number of available shows during peak hours

61. **How did CDNs support the launch of Microsoft Office 365 by ensuring faster download times for software packages?**

A) By storing all Office 365 updates at a single origin server

B) By caching Office 365 installation files at edge servers, speeding up download times for users across multiple regions

C) By compressing Office 365 software files

D) By limiting the number of users who can download the software at the same time

62. **What role did CDNs play in the success of YouTube's video-on-demand service?**

A) By compressing all video files

B) By caching video content at edge servers, reducing buffering and ensuring fast, reliable streaming for users worldwide

C) By limiting access to certain content

D) By restricting the resolution of videos during peak usage

63. **How did CDNs help with the high-speed delivery of online newspaper content like The Washington Post?**

A) By compressing articles

B) By caching articles, images, and videos at multiple edge servers to ensure quick load times for users around the world

C) By reducing the quality of images during peak hours

D) By limiting access to certain articles based on region

64. **Why did CDNs assist the U.S. government in handling large traffic volumes during the healthcare.gov launch?**

A) By limiting access to specific users

B) By caching frequently accessed pages and assets, ensuring faster load times and reducing server strain during high-traffic periods

C) By compressing all user data

D) By restricting access to certain forms

65. **How did CDNs improve the content delivery for online video platform, Youku, in China?**

A) By compressing videos

B) By caching videos and other media at edge servers, allowing for fast delivery even in regions with high internet traffic or slower connections

C) By restricting access to content in some regions

D) By storing all videos at a single origin server

66. **How did CDNs benefit large-scale media events like the Super Bowl broadcast in the U.S.?**

    A) By limiting the number of viewers per stream

    B) By caching live sports events and commercials at edge locations, providing seamless streaming and reducing latency during live broadcasts

    C) By compressing video feeds

    D) By reducing the number of simultaneous streams available

67. **Why did CDNs play a crucial role in helping the streaming service Hulu scale up during peak traffic events?**

    A) By limiting the number of available shows

    B) By caching video content at edge servers, reducing buffering and improving playback performance during high-demand events like premieres

    C) By reducing video resolution

    D) By restricting access to certain regions during high-traffic times

68. **How did CDNs help Twitter handle increased traffic during live events such as elections or sports games?**

    A) By limiting access to certain hashtags

    B) By caching tweets and media content at edge servers, ensuring faster load times and a smooth experience for users during peak events

    C) By compressing tweets and media

    D) By restricting access to certain users

69. **What advantage did CDNs provide to the online photo sharing platform, Instagram, during high-traffic periods?**

    A) By limiting access to certain photos

    B) By caching photos and videos at edge servers globally, reducing latency and ensuring smoother user experience across the world

    C) By compressing all photos

    D) By restricting image quality during peak times

70. **How did CDNs support the fast delivery of product images for e-commerce platforms like Etsy?**

    A) By compressing images

B) By caching product images, descriptions, and listings at edge servers, ensuring faster page load times and a better shopping experience for users worldwide

C) By reducing the number of product images

D) By limiting access to certain product categories

71. **How did Spotify improve its global music streaming service using a CDN?**

A) By limiting the number of songs per playlist

B) By caching music tracks and playlists at edge locations, ensuring faster access and smoother streaming for global users

C) By reducing the number of available music tracks

D) By compressing all song files

72. **How did Akamai's CDN assist Dropbox in delivering files to users around the world?**

A) By compressing all file data

B) By caching file downloads and uploads at edge locations to improve file transfer speeds and reduce latency for users globally

C) By limiting the size of uploaded files

D) By restricting access to certain file types

73. **How did CNN use a CDN to optimize the delivery of its live video news coverage during global events?**

A) By limiting the number of viewers per live broadcast

B) By caching live video streams at multiple edge locations, ensuring faster delivery and reduced latency for global viewers

C) By compressing video streams in real-time

D) By restricting access to certain regions during live coverage

74. **How did the online marketplace Alibaba use CDNs to scale its platform during peak shopping events like Singles' Day?**

A) By reducing the number of available products

B) By caching product pages, reviews, and checkout data at edge servers to handle massive traffic surges and ensure fast load times for users

C) By compressing all product images

D) By limiting access to certain products during peak periods

75. **Why did National Geographic implement a CDN to distribute high-definition video content on its website?**

A) By compressing HD videos

B) By caching HD video content at edge servers, ensuring faster load times and smooth playback for users around the world

C) By limiting access to HD videos

D) By reducing the resolution of videos during peak traffic times

76. **How did the CDN help with the performance of BBC's live sports streaming during major events like the Olympics?**

A) By compressing live video streams to reduce bandwidth usage

B) By caching live streams and video highlights at edge locations, ensuring faster and more reliable delivery to users worldwide

C) By limiting access to certain live events

D) By reducing the resolution of video streams based on user device

77. **How did the CDN support the global launch of a popular mobile app like Pokemon Go?**

A) By compressing in-app assets

B) By caching app data and user interactions at edge servers, ensuring fast app download times and minimizing latency for a global user base

C) By restricting the number of simultaneous logins per user

D) By limiting the number of regions where the app could be downloaded

78. **How did CDNs help Amazon Prime Video deliver its content efficiently to users worldwide?**

A) By compressing all video content

B) By caching content like movies and TV shows at multiple edge locations, ensuring fast streaming and minimal buffering for users around the globe

C) By limiting the resolution of streams during peak usage

D) By restricting access to certain video formats

79. **How did CDNs improve the performance of video-on-demand platforms like Netflix during peak hours?**

A) By limiting the number of viewers per show

B) By caching video content at edge servers, reducing latency and ensuring smooth streaming even during high-traffic periods

C) By compressing video files

D) By restricting access to certain movies or shows

80. **How did the CDN help improve user experience on a global scale for YouTube during major live events?**

A) By limiting access to certain streams

B) By caching live streams and videos at edge servers to ensure low-latency streaming and high-quality playback during global events like concerts and sporting events

C) By compressing all live streams

D) By reducing the video resolution for users with low internet speeds

81. **What role did CDNs play in assisting with the delivery of content for the online retail platform, Shopify?**

A) By compressing product images

B) By caching product pages, images, and checkout information at edge servers, improving load times for e-commerce sites and handling traffic spikes during sales events

C) By limiting the number of products on sale

D) By restricting the number of active users during peak traffic periods

82. **How did CDNs assist with the global performance of the online news platform, The Guardian?**

A) By compressing all images and articles

B) By caching articles, images, and videos at multiple edge servers, ensuring faster load times and smooth delivery of news content worldwide

C) By reducing the number of articles available during peak hours

D) By limiting access to content during high-traffic events

83. **Why did a CDN help with global performance for online streaming platforms like Twitch during esports tournaments?**

A) By limiting the number of viewers per stream

B) By caching video streams at edge locations, ensuring smooth and low-latency broadcasting for a global audience during large esports events

C) By reducing video quality during live events

D) By restricting access to specific game streams

84. **How did CDNs benefit the global content delivery for Adobe Creative Cloud?**

A) By compressing design files

B) By caching assets like creative tools and updates at edge servers, ensuring fast download times and a smooth experience for global users of Adobe software

C) By limiting the number of users who can access design assets

D) By reducing the quality of image and video assets during peak usage times

85. **How did CDNs assist with the high-speed delivery of large software packages like Windows updates for Microsoft?**

A) By limiting the number of downloads available

B) By caching update files at edge locations, ensuring faster and more reliable distribution of software updates to users worldwide

C) By compressing update files to reduce download size

D) By restricting the update availability to certain regions

86. **How did CDNs help with the global delivery of mobile app updates on platforms like the Apple App Store?**

A) By compressing all app updates

B) By caching app installation and update files at edge servers, improving download speeds and ensuring a smooth experience for users worldwide

C) By limiting the number of simultaneous downloads

D) By restricting access to updates during peak periods

87. **How did CDNs assist the global distribution of educational videos on platforms like Khan Academy?**

A) By compressing videos to reduce bandwidth

B) By caching educational videos at edge servers, ensuring faster load times and smooth playback for learners worldwide

C) By limiting access to some videos

D) By reducing video resolution during peak usage

88. **Why did CDNs help the delivery of content for the gaming platform, Epic Games Store?**

A) By restricting access to certain game files

B) By caching game downloads and updates at edge servers, reducing latency and ensuring faster download speeds for players globally

C) By compressing game files for faster downloads

D) By limiting the size of game files available for download

89. **How did CDNs improve the video streaming experience for mobile users on platforms like HBO Max?**

A) By limiting video streaming quality

B) By caching videos and streaming content at edge locations, ensuring fast and reliable delivery to mobile users worldwide, even during high-traffic periods

C) By reducing the number of available videos on the platform

D) By restricting access to mobile streams

90. **How did CDNs help the U.S. Department of Defense optimize its global delivery of secure data?**

A) By limiting access to certain files

B) By caching data securely at edge servers, ensuring fast and secure delivery of sensitive files to military personnel worldwide

C) By compressing all data files

D) By restricting access to sensitive files based on user role

91. **How did CDNs improve the performance of online marketplaces like eBay during global sales events?**

A) By limiting the number of available listings

B) By caching product images, listings, and checkout information at edge servers, improving load times and handling traffic surges during high-demand events

C) By compressing product images to reduce load times

D) By restricting the number of active users during sales

92. **How did the National Aeronautics and Space Administration (NASA) use a CDN for distributing large datasets?**

A) By compressing the datasets

B) By caching large scientific datasets at multiple edge servers, ensuring faster and reliable access to researchers and the public across the globe

C) By limiting the amount of data available for download

D) By restricting data access based on user location

93. **What was the role of a CDN in enhancing the performance of online ticketing platforms like Ticketmaster?**

A) By limiting the number of tickets available

B) By caching ticket information, venue details, and event schedules at edge locations, ensuring fast page load times and reducing congestion during high-demand events

C) By compressing all ticket images and event details

D) By restricting the number of ticket purchases per session

94. **Why did e-commerce platforms like Alibaba benefit from CDNs during global shopping events like Singles' Day?**

A) By reducing the number of available products

B) By caching product pages and shopping data at edge locations to handle massive traffic surges and ensure quick load times during high-demand periods

C) By compressing product descriptions and images

D) By restricting product access during peak hours

95. **How did CDNs enhance the delivery of 360-degree and VR content on platforms like Oculus?**

A) By compressing all VR content

B) By caching VR and 360-degree video content at edge servers, reducing latency and providing users with smooth playback experiences

C) By limiting access to VR content

D) By reducing the quality of VR videos

96. **How did Netflix use CDNs to optimize video streaming for users with varying internet speeds?**

A) By reducing video resolution for all users

B) By caching adaptive bitrate streams at edge locations, delivering video content based on user bandwidth and device capabilities

C) By compressing all video content

D) By restricting access to certain video qualities

97. **How did the streaming platform Disney+ handle global demand during the release of major content like "The Mandalorian"?**

A) By compressing video files for all users

B) By caching content at multiple edge servers, ensuring fast streaming and high-quality playback during high-traffic periods

C) By limiting the number of available episodes

D) By restricting access to content in certain regions

98. **How did a CDN improve the performance of e-learning platforms like Coursera during live sessions?**

A) By limiting the number of students per course

B) By caching course materials and live session streams at edge locations, ensuring fast and smooth delivery of content to students around the world

C) By compressing all video lectures

D) By restricting access to certain courses

99. **How did a CDN help optimize the delivery of interactive content for platforms like Buzzfeed?**

A) By limiting the number of interactive content pieces

B) By caching interactive media such as quizzes, videos, and polls at edge servers, ensuring faster load times and reducing latency during high traffic periods

C) By compressing interactive media

D) By restricting access to specific regions

100. **Why did the streaming service Peacock use CDNs for its content delivery?**

A) By compressing video files

B) By caching video streams at edge locations, ensuring smooth playback and reducing buffering for users across the globe, especially during peak usage times

C) By reducing the resolution of video streams

D) By limiting access to certain shows

The Core Concepts of CDN Architecture Answer

1. C	30. D	59. B
2. B	31. B	60. B
3. C	32. D	61. A
4. B	33. C	62. A
5. C	34. B	63. A
6. B	35. A	64. C
7. B	36. B	65. C
8. B	37. A	66. B
9. B	38. A	67. A
10. B	39. A	68. D
11. A	40. B	69. B
12. B	41. B	70. B
13. B	42. B	71. A
14. B	43. D	72. B
15. C	44. B	73. B
16. C	45. B	74. B
17. C	46. B	75. B
18. B	47. C	76. D
19. B	48. B	77. B
20. B	49. B	78. D
21. A	50. B	79. A
22. B	51. A	80. B
23. C	52. D	81. A
24. B	53. B	82. B
25. B	54. C	83. D
26. C	55. B	84. B
27. B	56. B	85. D
28. B	57. C	86. A
29. A	58. B	87. D

88. B   93. B   98. D

89. A   94. D   99. A

90. D   95. A   100.   B

91. B   96. A

92. D   97. A

CDN Performance and Optimization answer

1. A	29. C	57. B
2. B	30. A	58. A
3. D	31. A	59. D
4. A	32. B	60. A
5. B	33. A	61. D
6. D	34. A	62. B
7. A	35. A	63. B
8. A	36. A	64. B
9. D	37. A	65. D
10. C	38. A	66. A
11. A	39. A	67. A
12. A	40. A	68. D
13. B	41. A	69. D
14. A	42. D	70. A
15. D	43. C	71. A
16. B	44. A	72. B
17. A	45. B	73. D
18. D	46. A	74. A
19. C	47. B	75. D
20. D	48. B	76. B
21. A	49. A	77. A
22. A	50. A	78. D
23. B	51. A	79. A
24. D	52. B	80. A
25. A	53. A	81. A
26. C	54. A	82. B
27. A	55. B	83. A
28. B	56. A	84. A

85. B	91. A	97. A
86. A	92. A	98. B
87. A	93. A	99. A
88. A	94. A	100.　　　A
89. A	95. A	
90. A	96. A	

Advanced CDN Techniques answer

1. A	30. A	59. A
2. B	31. A	60. A
3. A	32. B	61. A
4. B	33. B	62. A
5. A	34. A	63. A
6. A	35. B	64. A
7. C	36. A	65. A
8. B	37. A	66. A
9. A	38. B	67. A
10. B	39. A	68. A
11. A	40. C	69. A
12. A	41. A	70. A
13. A	42. A	71. A
14. A	43. A	72. A
15. C	44. A	73. A
16. A	45. A	74. A
17. B	46. A	75. A
18. A	47. A	76. A
19. B	48. A	77. A
20. A	49. A	78. A
21. A	50. A	79. A
22. B	51. A	80. A
23. A	52. A	81. A
24. A	53. A	82. A
25. A	54. A	83. A
26. B	55. A	84. A
27. A	56. A	85. A
28. A	57. A	86. A
29. A	58. A	87. A

88. A	93. A	98. A
89. A	94. A	99. A
90. A	95. A	100. A
91. A	96. A	
92. A	97. A	

CDN Use Cases and Industry Applications answer

1. **B**	31. **B**	61. **B**
2. **B**	32. **B**	62. **B**
3. **B**	33. **B**	63. **B**
4. **B**	34. **B**	64. **B**
5. **B**	35. **B**	65. **B**
6. **B**	36. **B**	66. **B**
7. **B**	37. **B**	67. **B**
8. **B**	38. **B**	68. **B**
9. **B**	39. **B**	69. **B**
10. **B**	40. **B**	70. **B**
11. **B**	41. **B**	71. **B**
12. **B**	42. **B**	72. **B**
13. **B**	43. **B**	73. **B**
14. **B**	44. **B**	74. **B**
15. **B**	45. **B**	75. **B**
16. **B**	46. **B**	76. **B**
17. **B**	47. **B**	77. **B**
18. **B**	48. **B**	78. **B**
19. **B**	49. **B**	79. **B**
20. **B**	50. **B**	80. **B**
21. **B**	51. **B**	81. **B**
22. **B**	52. **B**	82. **B**
23. **B**	53. **B**	83. **B**
24. **B**	54. **B**	84. **B**
25. **B**	55. **B**	85. **B**
26. **B**	56. **B**	86. **B**
27. **B**	57. **B**	87. **B**
28. **B**	58. **B**	88. **B**
29. **B**	59. **B**	89. **B**
30. **B**	60. **B**	90. **B**

91. **B**	95. **B**	99. **B**
92. **B**	96. **B**	100. **B**
93. **B**	97. **B**	
94. **B**	98. **B**	

Case Studies of CDN Success answer

1. B	30. B	59. B
2. B	31. B	60. B
3. B	32. B	61. B
4. B	33. B	62. B
5. B	34. B	63. B
6. B	35. B	64. B
7. B	36. B	65. B
8. B	37. B	66. B
9. B	38. B	67. B
10. B	39. B	68. B
11. B	40. B	69. B
12. B	41. B	70. B
13. B	42. B	71. B
14. B	43. B	72. B
15. B	44. B	73. B
16. B	45. B	74. B
17. B	46. B	75. B
18. B	47. B	76. B
19. B	48. B	77. B
20. B	49. B	78. B
21. B	50. B	79. B
22. B	51. B	80. B
23. B	52. B	81. B
24. B	53. B	82. B
25. B	54. B	83. B
26. B	55. B	84. B
27. B	56. B	85. B
28. B	57. B	86. B
29. B	58. B	87. B

88. B	93. B	98. B
89. B	94. B	99. B
90. B	95. B	100. B
91. B	96. B	
92. B	97. B	

Made in United States
Orlando, FL
29 December 2024